# FUNCTIONAL FITNESS AT HOME

## ACKNOWLEDGMENTS

Thank you to my son, Christopher, for participating in our first book project. He is learning the steps to becoming a professional fitness trainer and is progressing well, but that always requires hard work. I wish him all the best. Thank you, Christopher Lowery!

I would also like to thank Firma Artzt for their cooperation with this third book project. It has been a great adventure. Thank you, Ludwig Artzt, GmbH.

A big thank-you goes to Meyer & Meyer Sport for a super collaboration and further business opportunities. Thank you, Martin Meyer.

—LAMAR TRAINING ACADEMY

# FUNCTIONAL FITNESS
## *At Home*

LAMAR AND CHRIS LOWERY

WITH THE COOPERATION
OF DAGMAR SCHOPEN
AND JULIAN BAKER

Meyer & Meyer Sport

British Library Cataloguing in Publication Data
A catalogue record for this book is available from the British Library

**Functional Fitness at Home**
Maidenhead: Meyer & Meyer Sport (UK) Ltd., 2017
ISBN: 978-1-7825-5121-8

© 2017 by Meyer & Meyer Sport (UK) Ltd.
Auckland, Beirut, Dubai, Hägendorf, Hong Kong, Indianapolis, Cairo, Cape Town,
Manila, Maidenhead, New Delhi, Singapore, Sydney, Teheran, Vienna
Member of the World Sports Publishers' Association (WSPA)
www.w-s-p-a.org
Printed by: Print Consult GmbH, Munich, Germany

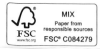

ISBN: 978-1-7825-5121-8
E-Mail: info@m-m-sports.com

# CONTENTS

# 1 INTRODUCTION– WHO IS LAMAR LOWERY?

When you see me, Lamar Lowery, you will inevitably think of an action figure that has come to life. As a six-foot, five-inch American model athlete with dual German–American citizenship, I am a constant commuter between the old and the new world. My job: personal trainer.

For 38 years, I have been training athletes, executives, and many other groups of people, using innovative training methods built around functional fitness. I was convinced from the start that a structured approach–a rather German mindset–determination and regular continued education, or rather, information, in the areas of training, tactics, and research can produce great results in the health and wellness industry. I have always considered this tenet in my own training.

## CAREER

- Benedict College 1984-1988/BA Sports Science
- Columbia Junior College/Midlands
- Technical College/Athletic scholarships
- 1986-1989 South Carolina Department of Lexington County Mental Health Hospital,
- Columbia, South Carolina
- Mental health specialist as a male nursing assistant
- 1989-1994 service in the U.S. Army
- Army master of physical fitness
- Instructor and master instructor
- Fitness Institute International, Inc./exercise science foundations course
- Fitness testing specialist course
- Functional training specialist course

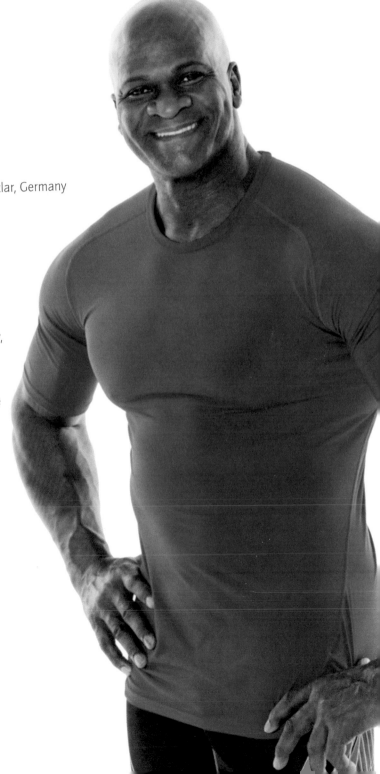

- Nutrition education and weight management specialist course
- Special populations/post-rehab specialist course
- Strength and conditioning specialist course
- CPTS
- Fascia training level 1
- Fascia training level 2

Functional Fascia Fortbildung, 2016
Fascia Research Summer School, 2016

## TRAINER ACTIVITY

- 1995-2000 World Sport West End, Wetzlar, Germany
- Maritim Hotel, Frankfurt, Germany
- Hilton Hotel, Frankfurt, Germany

## PERSONAL TRAINER

- 2000-2003 part-time coaching
- 2003-2005 Personal Training Company, Palm Beach, Florida
- HARMONY TRAINING WITH LAMAR
- 2005-2007 MS in Sales Representative Consulting & Training GmbH, Wetzlar, Germany

## PERSONAL TRAINER

2007 founding of the
Lamar Functional Training Academy

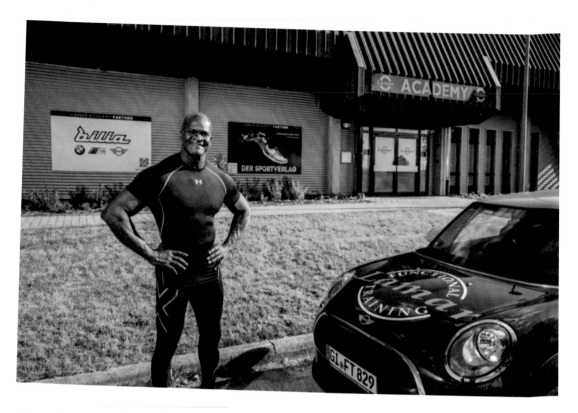

I have always dreamed of having my own training facility. For 15 years, I have been a successful personal trainer in Germany, have been working with the leaders of large companies as well as many celebrities, and have been a contributor to trade journals. Nine years ago, I founded the Lamar Functional Training Academy. My functional training is comprised of individual exercises that are specifically geared to the client's respective activities. My clients in Germany include the very busy Frankfurt executive as well as the successful business person from Gießen or the retiree who wants to improve his golf handicap.

To me, as a health professional, a good education, a well-trained eye, and lots of experience are the most important qualifications for the success of clients and trainers. Thanks to these foundations I am also able to help those recovering after an operation or injury to eliminate pain. Many people suffering from back pain feel fit, healthy, and resilient again after a specific workout with me. I live by my conviction: Targeted functional training is the best training for everyday life.

## The Functional Fitness Philosophy

"Preservation of health is a duty. However, few people seem to be conscious of such a concept as physical morality."

Although this quote is applicable today and might appear to have been written by a contemporary fitness evangelist, this is not the case. These words were spoken centuries ago by a Greek physician named Hippocrates—the father of medicine. Obviously, this historical figure valued health to the degree that he envisioned moral obligations extending beyond the physician and his professional commitment, a concept which we today know as the Hippocratic Oath.

What is physical morality? How does it relate to our present value systems? Should it be a part of our lives? And if so, would health education and promotion be able to effect behavioral change in this area? Answers to these questions lay the foundation for an understanding of our current health problems and their solutions.

By physical morality, Hippocrates meant that individuals had an ethical responsibility to take charge of their own health. Those who failed to maintain and preserve their health to the best of their abilities were shrinking their duties as citizens and, therefore, were guilty of immoral behavior. To the average American, this would undoubtedly seem a harsh definition, especially in our democratic society where we cherish our freedoms—even, perhaps, the freedom to neglect our health. It is likely that many would say that to choose to be unhealthy is one of our inalienable rights. But is it?

When we neglect our health, we become a tremendous burden to society. Nowhere is this more painfully evident than in America which has witnessed an outrageous explosion in healthcare costs of approximately $500 billion, or 11% of our GNP. Due to this astronomical expenditure, we are presently confronted with doubts about the stability of both Medicare and Medicaid.

As a result of our failure to adapt to the age of automation by programming physical activity and healthy eating into our lifestyles, Americans experience excessive degeneration and illness in later years. As a country, we are suffering the pitfalls of technological success. Labor-saving machines have created not only more leisure time, but also the sedentary lifestyle. Human bodies, built for rugged physical exertion, have become bloated and diseased with disuse. In the land of plenty, the motivation born of hard times has given way to indolence. The abundance of food has made every day a feast day and America the world's most overweight society. Even the miracles of modern medicine have done relatively little to prevent the increase of heart attacks, strokes, and senility caused by a diet too rich and a lifestyle too lacking in physical activity. Modern technology may keep people alive longer, but only a healthy lifestyle will ensure a vigorous, robust existence free of debilitation and multiple trips to the hospital.

Because of this self-neglect and the increased cost of medical care, health insurance premiums have risen to staggering heights. To date, unfortunately, insurance companies have not really differentiated between those who take care of themselves and those who do not. Consequently, the healthy who make few claims are paying similar rates to the unhealthy who utilize the healthcare system frequently.

Many people who take pride in their health and possess self-respect for their bodies take great offense at those who smoke, overeat, overdrink, use drugs, fail to exercise, and, in general, practice self-destruction. And well they should, for the unhealthy are a principle reason for the exceedingly high healthcare costs which must be borne by all.

As Hippocrates stated so long ago, perhaps everyone should recognize the moral imperative of good health. Or rather, everyone should make a philosophical commitment to good health within his or her value system. Maybe this is a duty, an obligation that befalls every member of society; for if one fails to live up to his physical capabilities, then he has placed an unfair burden on others. Expressed another way, when one neglects his health, he neglects not only his personal well-being but also the well-being of his family, his friends, his employer, and his country.

If health education and promotion are to facilitate the development of a broad-based value system of health in which we avoid becoming a burden to others, then we must establish an operative definition of *health*. Recognizing that individuals will always have varying definitions of health, there still ought to be a comprehensive concept that permits a degree of freedom but ensures that health habits are to the benefit of society, not its detriment.

Unfortunately, health is still primarily defined as just the absence of disease. Although a supposed fitness trend has been sweeping the country, most people pay only lip service to any real concept of health. We say there is nothing we value more than health; yet, in reality, there is nothing we abuse more than our health and well-being. Typically, we concern ourselves with our health only when it is in jeopardy. It is a tragedy that we emphasize sickness rather than optimal health; that we are concerned with not dying rather than really living; and that we fail to accept the challenge of life's greatest potential.

However, a few people today are redefining health as they begin to view this concept from a broader perspective. For these individuals, no longer is health just the absence of disease, but rather the wholesome lifestyle evidenced through vitality, productivity, and happiness. In fact, this positive view has been written into the preamble of the World Health Organization's constitution which reads: "Health is a state of complete physical, mental, and social well-being, not merely the absence of disease or infirmity."

This new definition of health is slowly making inroads into the American psyche through a number of different appellations which are currently receiving more attention. *Total fitness, holistic health, health enhancement*, and *lifestyle modification* are some of the more commonly used terms in describing this broad approach to the concept of health. Probably the most descriptive term which is slowly gaining general acceptance is that of *wellness*.

Much of the solution to our health problem is not only recognizing the perils of affluence, but more importantly, also redefining the good life and affirming the fact that we can be healthy and fit. To turn the health of this country around, the public must be awakened to its current unhealthy lifestyle and then be committed to refusing to allow this way of life to continue. As a nation, we must reconsider our goals through learning to value the quality of our lives as much as its material quantity.

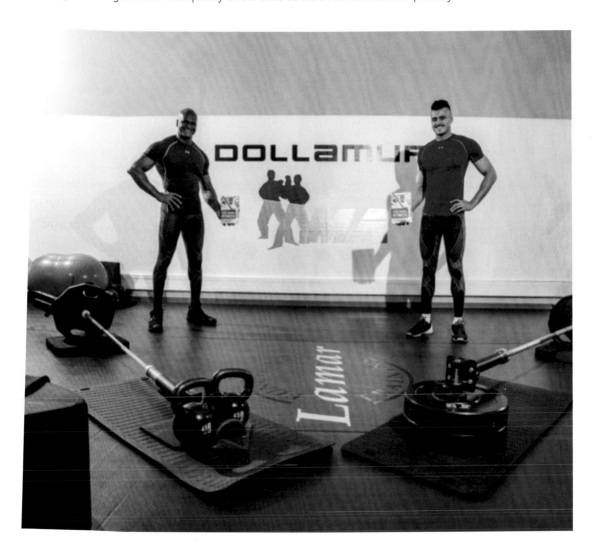

# 2 FUNCTIONAL TRAINING

Functional training is not new; rather, we have encountered it for several years, and currently it is probably one of the most overused terms in the fitness industry. An Internet search of functional training will produce 23,600,000 hits.

In the fitness industry, the market trend pendulum will swing heavily in a certain direction. Currently it has swung to the area of functional training. There was a time when many trainers used what I like to call the "Cirque de Soleil" training method. The philosophy behind this method excoriated any training exercise less complex than a one-armed shoulder press with a dumbbell while standing on one leg on a BOSU balance trainer as not functional and not suitable for everyday life. The problem with this philosophy is twofold. For one, the likelihood of executing a one-armed shoulder press with a weight while standing on one leg on an unstable surface is relatively low in everyday life, and, secondly, the more instability we add to an exercise, the smaller the load we can tolerate.

This type of training allows us to overload the central nervous system but hardly allows us to overload the musculature to create the necessary training stimulus—an example of a concept that could have some value but was overused. The reaction to this extreme philosophy was a big swing of the pendulum in the opposite direction. Suddenly the use of stability balls and balance boards in training was viewed in a negative light, and some trainers and therapists completely banished useful training aids from their sphere of activity.

While many people tend to believe that there is only one superior form of training and everything else that doesn't fit this philosophy is of no value, actually, there are and should be many different effective forms of training. Anything that helps us reach our goals should be used. What we mean by *functional fitness* is the ability to improve daily functionality through movement patterns that we humans use every day—simple, effective workouts without a safety net and false bottom.

The one-sided activities in our jobs and recreation often result in a general lack of movement along with poor posture, decreased fitness, and, thereby, lower quality of life. The current trend is "back to the roots," away from extreme sports and exaggerated weight loss and back to balanced exercise where the focus is on increased well-being and disease prevention.

Our functional training draws on tried and tested training principles and combines them in an efficient manner. It adopts the body's natural tasks, its movements and functions, and practices movement patterns from everyday life to balance body, spirit, and soul and to preserve that balance long-term.

The goal of functional training is to "wake up" the body and give it mobility for life. This is done through

- targeted movement of ideally all the body's muscles and joints,
- targeted movement and activation of the spine,
- activation of the neurological system,
- activation of the nervous system, and
- activation of the muscular system.

The exercises in our functional training program make people stronger, more powerful, and draw from many training philosophies. My long-time international experience in fitness training and ongoing exchange with personal trainers in the US make my concept unique. This book provides an insight into my world of functional fitness training.

# 2.1 DEFINITION

*Functional training* is a revolutionary training method from the US with ancient roots. Functional training can be labeled as the latest hype or as the catchphrase of the sports scene. At the same time, the content of this form of training is still hotly debated. The best way to define functional training is to take a closer look at the original meaning of the individual words.

*Function* can be defined as carrying out an action for which a person is specifically equipped or intended. Meaning, a function has a specific purpose. *Training*, on the other hand, denotes a complex process that induces an altered development by processing stimuli. You could say that functional training develops or practices movements the body was built for with the goal of achieving an altered, ideally improved, sense of well-being, meaning purposeful training. But purposeful is relative because it is always subject to the individual situation. Thus, we can train a mason so he is able to execute his activities of heavy lifting, bending, stretching, and diagonal reaching particularly effectively; while an older woman needs the necessary leg strength and coordination to walk up the stairs to her third-floor apartment; and the elite soccer player needs, next to speed, strength, and endurance, particularly good reaction ability and ball coordination. All of these factors cannot be viewed separately.

The human body is an extremely complex work of art. The constant interplay between different body systems and their individual parts enables the functions that define our lives. With its present-day construction adapted to its respective environment, the human body is the product of a long evolutionary process. We must, therefore, also allow individual scope for functional training—a scope that personal trainers use for the benefit of the client and to achieve the best-possible results.

In summary, functional training has the following characteristics:

- Everyday and sport specific

- Individual, yet still specific

- Versatile and varied

- Progressive

**With those characteristics, functional training follows five global principles:**

1. Integration, not isolation—Training complex movement sequences, meaning not just isolating individual muscles, but rather entire muscle chains the way they are used in everyday life.

2. Multidimensional bandwidth—Training movement patterns from daily life (everyday tasks, job, sports) that require the use of multiple joints on different planes.

3. Quality over quantity.

4. Using the body's own stabilizers, especially core stability, instead of external stabilizers such as chairs or benches.

5. Addressing correctable compensations and dysfunctions.

Body awareness and coordination are important parts of training within all these principles. Training must also emphasize muscle and joint mobility, areas that unfortunately still don't receive enough attention in some forms of training but are very important for good quality of life and injury prevention in sports.

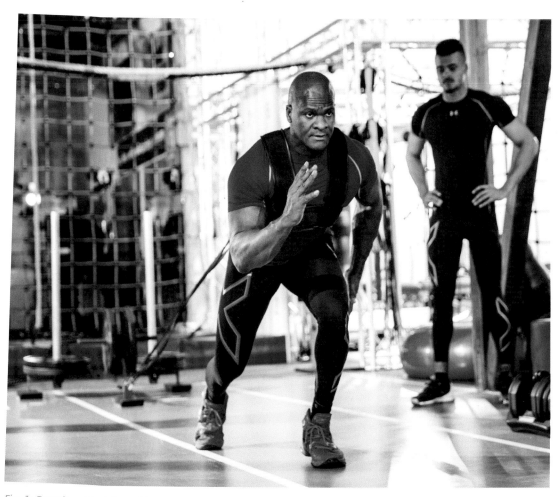

*Fig. 1: Functional training with Lamar*

## 2.2 PHILOSOPHY BEHIND COMPLETE TRAINING— FUNDAMENTALS OF FUNCTIONAL FITNESS

To understand complete training, we must examine the three main systems that essentially allow our bodies to function in our daily lives: the central nervous system, the nervous system, and the muscle system. Another system, the skeletal system, should also be taken into account.

These systems form a kind of symbiosis. A comparison from the realm of technology would be the car in which one important part cannot function without another. For instance, the engine cannot work without the fuel supply and ignition system, which in turn cannot work without electricity, and the cooling system is also crucial. Then there is the transmission, the chassis, wheels, and tires. But the body and windows as well as the entire interior make no sense without the previously mentioned systems and are what makes a car a car. If we removed all the technology and its interconnectedness, we would be left with the car's "nude body," the shell. We must, therefore, understand how important it is that each individual system functions, because each system becomes the problem of the whole if it does not function properly.

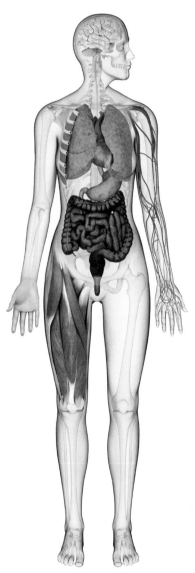

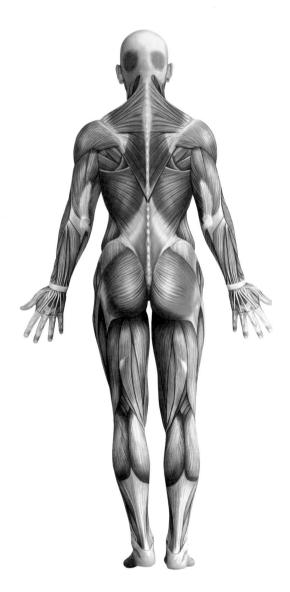

*Fig. 2: The central nervous system, the nervous system, and the musculature as central systems of the human body*

*Fig. 3: View of the human muscular system*

To keep this interplay intact, the individual organs in the human body must be connected directly or indirectly, much like the wires and parts of a car. The skeleton that lends the body support and shape makes such connections possible. Nearly all organs are in contact with each other and, at the same time, are protected through a framework of cartilage and bone, which is also the comprehensive network of the fascia. Vital substances such as red blood cells for oxygen transport and mineral salts are provided courtesy of through our bones. Moreover, lots of receptors in the fascia provide an extensive exchange of information.

## 2.3 MUSCULATURE

A more expansive chapter on anatomy, the individual muscle systems, and their functions could follow here. But since the focus of this book is training, I will instead refer to existing literature dedicated strictly to that topic and will only briefly address those areas important and relevant to practical training.

The skeleton of an adult human is comprised of approximately 206 individual bones that are connected by real or artificial joints. Our body possesses about 650 muscles without which we would not be able to move.

It is unlikely that such a large number of muscles within the "intelligent" human system developed solely for inactivity and rest. On the contrary, the human system is genetically constructed for movement and continuous loading. Our musculature weighs more than our bone frame (i.e., skeleton). While muscle makes up about 40% of our body weight, the skeleton is only 14%. The interplay of muscular, skeletal, and nervous systems makes human motion possible.

Each of our movements or postures requires activity of certain muscles. Muscle movements can only take place in conjunction with the nervous system and the brain. Our sensory organs allow us to perceive stimuli and sensations that are transmitted to the brain through the nervous system. It reacts with the appropriate orders that are then transmitted to the muscles through the nervous system. Each of these muscles is a separate organ consisting of skeletal muscle tissue, blood vessels, tendons, and nerves. Muscle tissue can also be found in the heart, in the digestive organs, and in the blood vessels. In these organs, muscles are responsible for the transport of substances throughout the body. They are constantly active. They cannot be controlled deliberately. The respiratory muscles are one example. We cannot deliberately release them from their activity. We must, therefore, note that there are three types of muscle tissue:

➡ Visceral or involuntary (smooth) muscles

➡ Heart muscle (special, striated muscle)

➡ Skeletal or voluntary (striated) muscles

## Visceral Musculature

*Visceral musculature* can be found in the organs—for instance, in the abdomen, in the colon, and in the blood vessels. It is the weakest muscle tissue, and it makes sure that organs contract in order to transport substances. Since visceral musculature cannot be controlled deliberately, it is also referred to as involuntary musculature. Due to its smooth, even appearance in microscopic images, it is also called smooth musculature. By contrast, heart and skeletal muscle is striped horizontally.

## Heart Muscle

The *heart muscle* makes sure that blood is pumped throughout the body. It cannot be controlled deliberately and is, therefore, an involuntary muscle. The heart muscle activates itself to contract. But the contraction frequency is regulated by hormones and signals from the brain. The natural heart pacemaker consists of heart muscle tissue that activates other heart muscle cells, prompting them to contract. Due to this self-activation, the heart muscle's function is considered autorhythmic, meaning its regulation is intrinsic.

The cells of the heart muscle are striped; when looking at them under a microscope, they appear to have light and dark bands. These light and dark bands are created by the arrangement of protein fibers in the cells. The horizontal stripes indicate that the muscle cell is very strong contrary to the visceral musculature.

## Skeletal Musculature

*Skeletal muscles* are the only voluntary muscles in the human body and are controlled deliberately. Every physical activity an individual consciously performs (e.g., talking, walking, or writing) requires skeletal muscle. A skeletal muscle contracts to bring parts of the body closer to the bone to which it is attached. Most skeletal muscles are attached to two bones across a joint so that the muscle can move parts of these bones closer together.

Many smaller precursor cells bundle together into long, straight, polynuclear fibers to form skeletal muscle cells. Like the heart muscle, skeletal muscles are striped horizontally, and skeletal muscle fibers are very strong. The name *skeletal muscle* stems from the fact that these muscles connect to the skeleton in at least one place.

## Relevance to Training—What Is Important?

When taking a closer look at the anatomical muscular system, it quickly becomes apparent that most muscles run diagonally or horizontally. The majority of trunk muscles (between the ischial tuberosity and the upper part of the sternum), more specifically 87.5%, run diagonally or horizontally. Their main function is movement. The following table shows the body is designed for rotational movement. Most trunk muscles are divided into vertical (no diagonal or rotational movement) and non-vertical (diagonal, horizontal, and rotational movement) muscle groups. Sometimes we differentiate between and refer to large and small muscles and the degree to which they participate in a rotation or support a rotation. Some leg muscles were included because they are connected to the pelvic floor and help to turn the body when it is on the ground.

When looking at the following table, you can see that the body's main function is rotation. Yet standard training concepts give little or no consideration to rotation.

*Table 1: Function and location of trunk muscles*

| MUSCLES | NONVERTICAL | VERTICAL |
|---|---|---|
| **Dorsal (back)** | | |
| Trapezius muscle (m. trapezius) | X | |
| Rhomboid muscle (m. rhomboideus major/minor) | X | |
| Latissimus dorsi (m. latissiumus dorsi) | X | |
| Erector spinae (m. erector spinae) | | X |
| Quadratus lumborum (m. quadratus lumborum) | X | |
| Gluteus maximus (m. gluteus maximus) | X | |
| Gluteus medius (m. gluteus medius) | X | |
| Gluteus minimus (m. gluteus minimus) | X | |
| Tensor fascia latae (m. tensor fasciae latae) | | X |
| Hip rotator muscles | X (6x) | |

| MUSCLES | NONVERTICAL | VERTICAL |
|---|---|---|
| Ventral (abdominal) | | |
| Pectoralis major (m. pectoralis major) | X | |
| Pectoralis minor (m. pectoralis minor) | X | |
| Serratus anterior (m. serratus anterior) | X | |
| External oblique muscle (m. obliquus externus abdominis) | X | |
| Internal oblique muscle (m. obliquus internus abdominis) | X | |
| Rectus abdominis (m. rectus abdominis) | | X |
| Transverse abdominal muscle (m. transversus abdominis) | X | |
| Psoas (m. psoas) | X | |
| Iliacus muscle (m. iliacus) | X | |
| Sartorius muscle (m. sartorius) | X | |
| Rectus femoris muscle (m. rectus femoris) | | X |
| Abductors | X (4x) | |
| Pectineus muscle (m. pectineus) | X | |
| Gracilis muscle (m. gracilis) | X | |
| Total | 28 pairs = 56 | 4 pairs = 8 |
| | % rotator muscles = 87.5% | |

The spiral is a universal element of our locomotor system. Our body is built based on the same functional principles. Therefore, nearly all training should include rotation as an important function.

**Complexity in Training:**

1. Posture
2. Coordination
3. Balance
4. Biomechanical axis
5. Speed
6. Strength components
7. Flexibility
8. Endurance

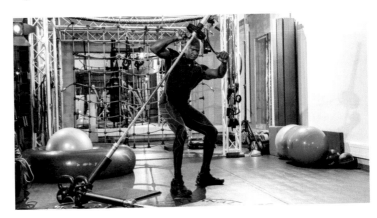

# 2.4  SKELETAL SYSTEM

The skeletal system is yet another of the systems that give the body life. Contrary to other living organs, bones are solid and strong, but they have their own blood and lymph vessels as well as nerves. Bones consist of two different types of tissue:

- Compact bone tissue: This sturdy, compact tissue forms the outer layer of most bones and the sheath of long bones, such as in the arms and legs. Nerves and blood vessels can be found in this tissue.

- Sponge-like bone tissue: This tissue consists of smaller trabeculae with red bone marrow located in between. It is found at the ends of long bones (e.g., the head of the femur) and inside other bones.

A fully-grown human body has 206 bones of which nearly 50% are located in the hands and feet. Joints or interstices connect the bones to each other and lend our bodies stability and protection for all internal organs. We differentiate between fibrous, or osseous, joints that move very little or not at all and true joints with different ranges of motion, depending on the type of joint.

Many joints can move on all three planes simultaneously (see the following table). For instance, a joint can be flexed, pulled toward the body, and internally rotated, all at the same time. Even the small joints in the ankle complex can perform movements that we may not even be aware of. The following table will help us to better understand functional movements.

*Table 2: Joint planes of motion*

| SAGITTAL PLANE/VERTICAL—BACK-TO-FRONT MOTION | |
| --- | --- |
| **JOINT** | **MOTION** |
| Hip | Flexion/extension |
| Knee | Flexion/extension |
| Ankle | Dorsal flexion/plantar flexion |
| Lower ankle joint | Dorsal flexion/plantar flexion |
| Midtarsal joint | Dorsal flexion/plantar flexion |
| **FRONTAL PLANE—LEFT-TO-RIGHT MOTION** | |
| **JOINT** | **MOTION** |
| Hip | Abduction/adduction |
| Knee | Abduction/adduction |
| Ankle | — |
| Lower ankle (subtalar joint) | Inversion/eversion |
| Midtarsal joint | Inversion/eversion |
| **TRANSVERSE PLANE—ROTATIONAL MOTION** | |
| **JOINT** | **MOTION** |
| Hip | External/internal rotation |
| Knee | — |
| Ankle | — |
| Lower ankle (subtalar joint) | — |
| Midtarsal joint | — |

| PRONATION | | | |
|-----------|--------|--------|-----------|
| JOINT | SAGITTAL | FRONTAL | TRANSVERSE |
| Hip | Flexion | Adduction | Internal rotation |
| Knee | Flexion | Abduction | Internal rotation |
| Ankle | Dorsal/Plantar flexion | – | Adduction/abduction |
| Lower ankle | – | Eversion | Adduction |
| Midtarsal joint | Dorsal flexion | Inversion | Abduction |
| SUPINATION | | | |
| JOINT | SAGITTAL | FRONTAL | TRANSVERSAL |
| Hip | Extension | Abduction | External rotation |
| Knee | Extension | Adduction | External rotation |
| Ankle | Dorsal/Plantar flexion | – | Adduction/abduction |
| Lower ankle | – | – | Adduction |
| Midtarsal joint | Plantar flexion | – | Adduction |

## Relevance to Training—What Is Important?

The joints are the human body's weak spot for anatomical reasons. Stability, mobility, and muscular control of joints should, therefore, be taken into account during training. The joint-encompassing muscles form a kind of protective wall that, with good neuromuscular control, can minimize or even prevent injuries.

## 2.5 CENTRAL NERVOUS SYSTEM

The *central nervous system* consists of the brain, spinal cord, and a complex neuronal network. This system is responsible for transmitting, receiving, and interpreting information from all parts of the body. The nervous system monitors and coordinates the function of internal organs and reacts to changes in the environment. It can be divided into two parts: the *central nervous system* and the *peripheral nervous system*.

The *central nervous system (CNS)* is the nervous system's processing center. It receives information from the peripheral nervous system and transmits information to the peripheral nervous system. The two main organs of the CNS are the brain and spinal cord. The brain processes and interprets sensory information transmitted by the spinal cord.

## 2.6 PERIPHERAL NERVOUS SYSTEM

The peripheral nervous system is a complex network of nerves and cells that transport messages to the brain and spinal cord and from the brain and spinal cord to other parts of the body. The peripheral nervous system consists of the somatic and vegetative nervous systems. Neuromuscular control has a major impact on movement quality.

### Relevance to Training—What Is Important?

An interruption can result in the incorrect or inefficient execution of movements. In the long term, these can be performance limiting or even lead to injuries. With sensorimotor training, this can often be prevented.

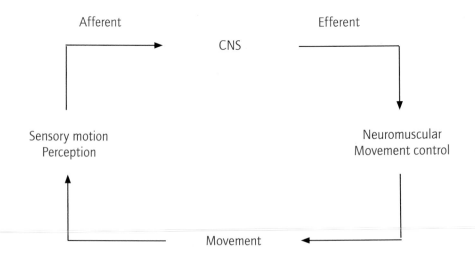

*Fig. 4: Simplified illustration of the sensorimotor regulatory circuit as per Bruhn and Gollhofer (2001, p 66)*

# 2.7 WHAT CAN FUNCTIONAL TRAINING ACCOMPLISH?

We have discussed functional training, but is this form of training just another "path to fitness" we must negotiate, or is it worth making a long-term commitment to our training and making it a part of our training practice? After 14 years working as a trainer, I am convinced that incorporating functional training into our current training practice is one of the most important steps toward basic fitness and health. Anyone who thinks he can be successful without factoring in health is wrong. Physical training does not only affect the muscles but also well-being and performance capacity. Endurance, properly dosed strength, and flexibility are the cornerstones of physical performance. Traditional weightlifting usually only focuses on one muscle per exercise, whereas a functional exercise can work multiple body regions and, thereby, muscle chains.

In my opinion, the most relevant positive effects of personalized functional training are

- increased (inner) strength,

- endurance,

- improved, optimized basic stability along with flexibility (mobility),

- increased quality of life and balance, and

- improved body awareness.

These improvements result in increased performance capacity and decreased susceptibility to stress—important building blocks that all of us would like to list on the asset side of life. Functional training makes muscles, fascia, and joints healthier and more stable, and just like we brush our teeth every day, we should do the same for our bodies and "remove the rust" through functional training.

Functional training works the muscles on different planes and, thus, from different angles. This targets stabilizing as well as fixator muscles. Gym equipment is preset and only allows the body to move within the preset angles and planes. In addition, the upper and lower body are often trained separately, which does not take into account the trunk as a stabilizing waypoint. Multiplane exercises are more complex and more accurately imitate the movements we perform in everyday life.

An easy way to integrate functional training into fitness training is to write down what your daily activities are as well as what possible physical challenges you may have. Have you noticed that your legs and back hurt at the end of your workday because you are constantly sorting binders and lifting them from the floor to your desk or placing them on shelves? Then that should be the first body region you work on. Examples of functional movements that use multiple joints and muscle chains are

- multidirectional lunges,

- standing bicep curls, and

- step-ups with weights.

Multidirectional lunges prepare the body for different everyday activities, such as vacuuming or yard work. In doing so, the lunge is not just performed in a forward direction, but in many different directions at various angles. It is recommended to start with exercises that use only your own body weight for physical loading. Weights and resistance can be integrated into the exercises as the fitness level increases.

## Benefits of Functional Training

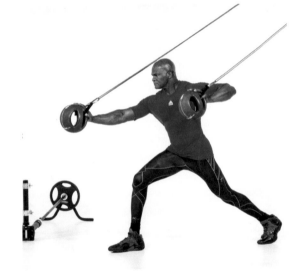

- Increase muscular strength

- Increase muscular endurance

- Increase muscle recruitment

- Decrease risk of injury

- Increase speed

- Decrease risks of disease and osteoporosis

- Develop lean muscle mass

- Lose weight

- Feel good

## How to Gain Benefits of Functional Training

The only entirely functional activity is the actual activity you are training for. You must train to enhance the coordinated working relationship between the nervous and muscular systems. The primary goal of functional training is to transfer the improvements in strength achieved in one movement to enhance the performance of another movement by affecting the entire neuromuscular system.

To increase the *transfer effect*, it is as critical to train the specific movement as it is to train the muscles involved in the movement. The highest transfer effects are movements that are essentially similar to the actual movement in coordination, type of muscular contraction, speed of movement, and range of motion.

Optimizing performance training requires optimal strength, power performance, and optimal stabilization, particularly core stabilization.

**Functional core training benefits:**

- Improves dynamic postural control.

- Ensures muscle balance.

- Provides intrinsic stability for lumbo–pelvic–hip complex, which allows for optimum neuromuscular efficiency of the rest of the kinetic chain.

Fitness training has really evolved over the last 38 years. It seems like only a few years ago, all I was doing was going to the gym, using machines for weight training, and hitting a couple of aerobics classes. But now I train frequently with different tools because it is fun to challenge myself to see how well I can perform.

These days, it is normal to be confused when determining which avenue you should take to get in shape. So take your time and learn with a trained professional. Take steps to do well in your training because there are so many different functional movement tools out there, and most fitness professionals have all the following available:

Yoga (vinyasa, ashtanga, hatha, bikram, hot vinyasa, jivamukti)

- Bootcamp

- Weight training

- Interval training

- Suspension training

- Kettlebell training

- Spinning

- Cardio equipment (stepmills, ellipticals, treadmills, VersaClimbers, exercise bikes, rowers)

- Battle rope training

- Swimming

## Determining Which Method Is Best for You

The first question to ask yourself is this: **What outcome do I want?** Do you want to improve body composition? Do you want to improve overall functionality and movement? Do you want to improve cardiovascular health?

Once you have the answer to this, you have a place to start. Now, I'm not saying you can't work on all three at the same time, but to help get you targeted and focused, I've broken it down as follows:

## Improving Body Composition

To improve body composition, you have to resistance train. Resistance training raises you BMR—basal metabolic rate—which is the amount of fat calories your body burns while at rest. Your BMR is higher during rest after weight training than after cardio alone, so you can see why resistance training is so crucial. Some great tools to use when resistance training are

- weights,

- kettlebells,

- cables,

- bands, and

- body weight.

## Improving Functionality and Movement

This is for the individual who feels like he is not moving as well as he used to, which makes up the majority of the clientele that I see. Let's face it, sitting in a chair eight hours a day will make anyone feel stiff. There are excellent methods to help improve functionality and movement. First, you should go through a functional movement screening or a specific assessment. Any good strength coach or physical therapist can run you through this. You will then be able to determine what your weak points are and correct those. If you do not have access to a specific screening, then there are some different methods you can follow:

- Yoga

- Pilates

- Gyrotonics

- Standard stretching methods

## Improving Cardiovascular Health

A basic method for improving cardiovascular health is for three days out of your week choose one activity from the following:

- Running

- Swimming

- Biking

- Paddleboarding

- Hiking

- Battle ropes

- Spinning

- Climbing regular stairs

- Using cardio equipment (stepmill, elliptical, treadmill, VersaClimber, exercise bike, rowing machine)

On day 1, pick something that you're able to do at high intensity for a short period of time—in other words, for 10 minutes or less. On day 2, do something at a medium intensity for up to 20 minutes. On day 3, choose something you can maintain for 30 to 60 minutes at a very slow, easy pace. This is a very broad approach, but it's great for the beginner.

At the end of the day, training has got to be enjoyable. Even my professional athletes who do this for a living have to keep things fun and interesting. So pick a goal and get focused, but always remember to have fun!

Now, let us have a look at what fitness type you are and what type you would like to become.

# 2.8 THREE FITNESS PHASES FOR BUILDING MUSCLES

If your goal is to build lean muscle mass, improve your strength, and define your body, then you have to train smarter, not harder. You can build a muscular physique naturally by following a phase-based approach: foundation phase, hypertrophy phase, and firming phase. You must balance what you like to do with what your body requires to grow and what it needs to recover from your workouts. If your goal is to improve your muscle mass, plan to progressively challenge the body by using these three phases of training.

## What You Should Know Before You Start

Each workout should last about 45 minutes to 1 hour, including a proper warm-up and cool-down. If you are new to using weights, begin with a full-body routine, three days a week. Each phase can last two to four weeks. Start with a higher number of repetitions and lower resistance, and gradually decrease the number of repetitions and increase the resistance as you progress. Begin with a variety of exercises, such as squats, chest presses, dumbbell rows, dumbbell shoulder presses, and exercises for the core and arms. Eating for muscle size is no different than eating for health; you just need more of everything. Eat a diet rich in vegetables and fruits, whole grains, and at least 1.0 to 1.5 grams of protein/kg of body weight. A whey protein supplement can be used in a shake or sprinkled on cereal to help your protein intake requirements.

## Phase 1: Foundation

The first phase of any resistance training program should build the foundation of strength, endurance, and the integrity of joints and other structures. This foundation phase focuses on circuit training, providing both a muscular and aerobic benefit. As you finish the first set of the first exercise, move immediately to the next exercise and so on until all exercises are complete. Rest 60 seconds, and repeat circuit for remaining sets. Use a moderate weight that you can lift with little discomfort.

## Phase 2: Hypertrophy

Once you build the foundation, you can challenge the muscles to grow. Hypertrophy is the term used to describe an increase in the size of a muscle. This is the phase that people quickly turn to when wanting to improve their physique. Many studies have shown that the 8- to 12-repetition range helps build the greatest amount of muscle mass along with producing the highest levels of growth hormone—a hormone that keeps the body young, vibrant, and healthy and fosters lean muscle growth. Use a challenging weight that makes every last repetition difficult. Unlike the foundation phase, you complete all sets of the first exercise before moving on to the second exercise, and so on. Rest period for this phase is one to two minutes.

## Phase 3: Firming

You have built a solid foundation, increased the size of your muscles, and now it is time to firm and tone your body. Lifting heavier weights is the next natural progression to firming the muscles. Choose a weight that challenges the final repetition. This phase is designed in a vertical format, with all exercises listed one beneath the other. Work your way down the list and complete the first set of all exercises, resting 60 to 120 seconds between sets before starting again from the top of the list and completing the remaining sets.

You can build a muscular physique naturally by following a phase-based approach. Adding cardiovascular training two to three times per week for 20 to 30 minutes at a moderate pace will also help burn fat and improve muscle definition.

*Table 3: Three fitness phases for muscle training*

| PHASE | NUMBER OF EXERCISES | NUMBER OF SETS | REPETITION RANGE | REST BETWEEN SETS (SECONDS) |
|---|---|---|---|---|
| Foundation | 3-4 | 8-10 | 15-20 | 60 |
| Hypertrophy | 4-5 | 6-8 | 8-12 | 60-90 |
| Firming | 3-5 | 6-8 | 5-7 | 60-120 |

# 2.9 INTEGRATED FITNESS TRAINING

*Integrated fitness training* is a model designed for the fitness enthusiast who has different goals in mind.

Understanding the structured concept is the foundation. The functional movement and resistance training phases are logical movement-based exercise programs and modifications that can be used to train for stability and mobility. In other words, this type of integrated fitness training improves postural imbalances as well as trains for speed, agility, quickness, and power for improved athletic performance. Furthermore, a new systematic approach to cardiorespiratory training can be used to reach any unique goals for health, fitness, or performance in endurance competitions.

Integrated fitness training also has a cardiovascular structure with four cardiorespiratory training phases:

- Phase 1: Aerobic-based training

- Phase 2: Aerobic efficiency training

- Phase 3: Anaerobic endurance training

- Phase 4: Anaerobic power training

Each phase has a primary training focus designed to facilitate specific physiological adaptations to exercise. Not every person starts in phase 1 because everyone has a unique entry point into the cardiorespiratory training phases based upon his or her current health, fitness, and goals. By using the assessment and programming tools in each phase, you can develop individualized cardiorespiratory programs that allow you to progress from being sedentary to training for performance in endurance events, if you wish. While most exercisers will not go through this full progression, it is empowering to have the tools to provide these long-term training solutions.

Programming in each phase is based on three training zones. The exercise intensities in each zone are based on individual-specific intensity markers that include heart rate (HR) at the first and second ventilatory thresholds (VT1 and VT2), the talk test, and ratings of perceived exertion (RPE).

Traditional intensity markers such as percentages of maximal HR (%MHR), HR reserve (%HRR), or $VO_2$ reserve (%$VO_2$R) are not the recommended methods for monitoring cardiorespiratory exercise intensity because they require actual measurement of MHR or $VO_2$max to provide accurate individualized data for programming. Most individuals do not have the equipment to assess $VO_2$max, and there is little or no reason to find your actual MHR unless $VO_2$max is also being assessed.

As such, anyone using these traditional intensity markers must estimate MHR and VO2max using equations with large standard deviations. Exercise guidelines based upon predicted MHR or VO2max can help you reach your goals, but these guidelines leave a lot of room for error and do not account for each person's unique metabolic response to exercise.

## Fitness Testing

Once you have been thoroughly screened and cleared for exercise, the next step is fitness testing. There are three reasons to test fitness:

1. To acquire education about your fitness status in relation to health standards for individuals of the same age and gender.

2. To provide data that will help you develop exercise programming for the different components of fitness.

3. To collect baseline data against which future testing data may be compared.

Gaining initial education of your health status is very important from a motivational standpoint. More importantly, however, is follow-up testing, which provides feedback about how you are progressing. Reinforcing your efforts gives you the taste of success which is essential for maintaining enthusiasm for ongoing training.

Prior to fitness testing, you should receive instructions on how to prepare for the various tests that will be administered. Explicit instructions are necessary to ensure the validity and accuracy of the data. In addition to not smoking within three hours of testing, you should also be instructed not to ingest food, alcohol, or caffeine. Besides appropriate attire, it is also important that you are well rested and have not exercised within the past 12 hours.

# 2.10 MORE FUNCTIONAL PROGRAMMING

**GENERAL STRENGTH** = Developed with your standard resistant training modalities (e.g., weight training, bodyweight exercises). General strength training does not mimic any specific activity movement. The main objective of this training phase is to create anatomical adaptions geared toward increasing maximum strength and work volume. Cleans, squats, shoulder presses, and bench presses are examples of exercises used to develop general strength.

**SPECIFIC STRENGTH** = Enhanced by exercises that closely resemble the actual mechanics of athletic movements. Many of the exercises used in the specific strength phase have been classified as functional exercises. This training phase begins the process of transferring general strength to a more specific function. Basic medicine ball throws and plyometrics are examples of specific strength exercises.

**EXACT SPECIFIC STRENGTH** = Optimize the transfer of general and specific strength to the target activity. This training phase tries to closely mimic target activity movements marked for improvement to their exact speed, load, and mechanics. Hitting a blocking sled, throwing a weighted ball, swinging a weighted bat, single-leg reaches, and band-resisted activity are examples of exact specific strength exercises.

**ACTIVE RECOVERY** = This allows the body to heal and regenerate from the training or competition. Active recovery is, by far, more effective then total rest. Cross-training and involvement in active hobbies are excellent approaches to take during recovery periods.

## Benefits of Regular Physical Activity and Exercise

- Improvement in cardiovascular and respiratory function

  - Increased maximal oxygen uptake due to both central and peripheral adaptations
  - Lower minute ventilation at a given submaximal intensity
  - Lower myocardial oxygen cost for a given absolute submaximal intensity
  - Lower heart and blood pressure at a given submaximal intensity
  - Increased capillary density in skeletal muscle
  - Increased exercise threshold for the accumulation of lactate in the blood
  - Increased exercise threshold for the onset of disease signs or symptoms (e.g., angina pectoris, ischemic ST-segment depression, claudication)

➤ Reduction in coronary artery disease risk factors

- Reduced resting systolic/diastolic pressures
- Increased serum high-density lipoprotein cholesterol and decreased serum triglycerides
- Reduced total body fat, reduced intra-abdominal fat
- Reduced insulin needs, improved glucose tolerance

➤ Decreased mortality and morbidity
- Primary prevention (i.e., interventions to prevent an acute cardiac event
1. Higher activity and fitness levels are associated with lower death rates from coronary artery disease.
2. Higher activity and fitness levels are associated with lower incidence rates for combined cardiovascular diseases, coronary artery disease, colon cancer, and type 2 diabetes.

- Secondary prevention (i.e., interventions after a cardiac event to prevent another)
1. Based on meta-analyses (pooled data across studies), cardiovascular and all-cause mortality are reduced in post-myocardial infarction patients who participate in cardiac rehabilitation exercise training, especially as a component of multifactorial risk factor reduction.
2. Randomized controlled trials of cardiac rehabilitation exercise training and all-cause mortality are reduced in post-myocardial infarction patients.

**Other postulated benefits:**

➤ Decreased anxiety and depression

➤ Enhanced feeling of well-being

➤ Enhanced performance of work, recreational, and sport activities

The purpose of fitness assessments is to gather baseline data and to provide a basis for developing goals and effective exercise programs. Gathering and evaluating various pieces of information provides a broader prospective of your fitness levels. The process and the data collected assist in identifying potential areas of injury and reasonable starting points for recommended intensities and volumes of exercise based on those goals and fitness outcomes. The data helps to classify your resistance training status.

# FUNCTIONAL FITNESS AT HOME

The following breaks down how to train based on your resistance status.

## Training Status

1.  Beginner (unfit)

2.  Intermediate (moderately fit)

3.  Advanced (fit)

## Current Program

1.  Not training or just began training (unfit)

2.  Currently training (moderately fit)

3.  Training more than one year (advanced, fit)

## Training Age

1.  < 2 months (unfit)

2.  2-6 months (moderately fit)

3.  1+ year (advanced, fit)

## Frequency (Per Week)

1.  < 1-2 (unfit)

2.  < 2-3 (moderately fit)

3.  3-4+ (advanced, fit)

## Training Stress

1.  None or low (unfit)

2.  Medium (moderately fit)

3.  High (advanced, fit)

# 2.11 What Is Yoga?

The term *yoga* originates from the Sanskrit word, YUI. It is often translated as harnessing, linking, or joining. Yoga is about controlling the erratic mind through consciousness to achieve holistic personal development.

It is difficult to date the origins of yoga since yoga knowledge was passed down secretly and orally in the form of rhythmic verses. The techniques were passed on from teacher to student. Originating in India, the first written records about yoga are mentioned in the Upanishads, a collection of Hindu philosophical writings from around 600 BC. Artistic depictions on signets found in northern India date back much further. The Yogic journey is at least 3,500 years long. The famous and systematic representations of yoga philosophy still relevant today, the Patanjali Yoga Sutras, originated during the classical yoga period. Little is known about Patanjali the person, not even the exact dates of when he lived, though records suggest somewhere between 300 BC and 300 AD. He initially mentions the complex system of yoga in his 195 Yoga Sutras. Here he describes the eightfold path, or eight arms, of Patanjali as a practice that must be pursued step by step.

They eight arms are:

- Yama (external discipline),

- Niyama (internal discipline),

- Asana (postures),

- Pranayama (breathing),

- Pratyahara (restraining the senses),

- Dharana (concentration),

- Dhyana (meditation), and

- Samadhi (becoming one, enlightenment).

The path of classical yoga consists of eight parts or steps. The first five steps describe the external path, and the final three steps describe the internal path. In the western world, many people think of yoga as an exclusively physical practice (Asana). But, in fact, this is only one of eight steps. For most people starting the practice of yoga, it seems easier to initially focus on the physical aspects, such as flexibility, health, or muscle tone. The physical traditions, therefore, make it easier to enthuse yoga beginners.

The Patanjali Sutras quickly drive home that yoga is not an athletic technique, but rather a way to bring mind, spirit, and body into unison. At the very beginning of his remarks, Patanjali defines the purpose of yoga: "Yogas citta-vritti-nirodah." Yoga is the internal state during which the emotional–spiritual processes come to rest. This millennia-old Indian technique that encompasses a number of mental and physical exercises as well as meditation has arrived in the midst of our western society. It is interesting that Patanjali says little about the physical practice (Asana) of yoga. In Sutra 2.46, he simply writes that the seated posture should be firm and comfortable ("sthira-sukham-āsanam"). This implies that what we think of as yoga today merely served as preparation for a meditation practice.

Many different styles of yoga have developed over time, often with a separate philosophy and practice. Some meditative forms of yoga focus on mental concentration, others on the physical practice (Asana) and deliberate breathing (Pranayama), while other forms emphasize asceticism. Today, yoga is mostly used to relax, to improve flexibility, and to decrease stress.

As a relaxation technique, yoga practices generally pursue a holistic approach intended to bring body, mind, and spirit into unison. In addition, yoga can help bring balance to an unbalanced lifestyle. It is, therefore, important to practice with some regularity. Particularly in western countries, yoga is often taught in teaching units. Such a unit combines Asana, phases of deep relaxation, as well as meditation.

There are many different yoga traditions. One of the most well known is Hatha Yoga, which is also the most popular style of yoga in the western world. It emphasizes physical alignment. Many other styles of yoga have developed from this and other traditional forms. For instance, the form of yoga developed by Swami Sivananda (1887-1963) has a more holistic approach, emphasizing deep relaxation and meditation next to physical and breathing exercises. The yoga instructor Iyengar (1918-2014) established a style of yoga that focuses on participation in and precision of yoga poses. Typical for this popular style of yoga is the use of blocks or straps. The challenging form of Ashtanga Yoga, which teaches Vinyasa (flowing exercises) and a particular breathing technique (Ujjayi breath), is also rooted in Hatha Yoga.

*Bikram Yoga*, developed by the yoga master of the same name, is practiced at approximately 104 °F and with high humidity. It consists of a specific sequence of Asana and two Pranayama techniques. *Kundalini Yoga*, established by Yogi Bhajan (1929-2004), consists of more than 1,500 practices that can be static as well as dynamic, very meditative, but also invigorating and stimulating. This type of yoga is very diverse and offers the participant a huge variety of options. It is also referred to as the yoga of awareness or the yoga of energy. There are several other yoga traditions worth mentioning, but that would go beyond the scope of this book. In principle, almost anyone can do yoga because it is not about performance or perfectionism, but simply about the practice. Physical limitations are not an impediment because many of the exercises can be adapted to the participant with the aid of assistive equipment. Highlighted here are just a few of the possible benefits of yoga:

- Strengthens the immune system

- Decreases back pain

- Reduces neck and shoulder tension

- Strengthens the parasympathetic nervous system

- Has a positive effect on heart and lungs

- Stimulates the endocrine system

- Improves sleep disorders

- Improves physical fitness

- Increases self-confidence

- Improves stress management

- Increases concentration

- Improves blood values

By now there are many international studies on the subject of yoga that, for instance, make it possible for conventional medicine to use and recommend yoga to enhance health. To date, western science has been unable to prove all the benefits of yoga. But that does not mean it isn't effective.

# 3 EXERCISES

The average person isn't terribly unhealthy and unfit but is ready to start exercising regularly. He might already run or bike but has never done any strength training.

So it is extremely important to have a certified professional that will assist in proper training structures as well as training in general when it comes to knowing proper form, learning how to train slow, and understanding how correct movement feels (this is also helped by training in front of mirrors). Knowing how to breathe correctly and being aware of your surroundings are also important to learn when beginning training. It is the job of the trainer to make sure the exerciser is using the correct training gear and is also mentally and physically prepared for the new demands placed on the body.

The fitness enthusiast has been exercising regularly but wants to step it up. To him, it is important to improve his performance and reach a new fitness level. For example, triathletes exercise at an entirely different level from most other fitness enthusiasts or athletes because their sport requires lengthy training prior to competition. Triathletes must train for all three endurance activities and understand how to manage their energy; they must be able to transition from one activity to another as smoothly as possible; and they must understand how to proceed on fatigued muscles. So this particular fitness enthusiast has different needs from, for instance, a running enthusiast.

Because the training needs are different for the individual based on fitness goals, the following workouts have been categorized based on different sports and activities, including stability exercises for runners, cyclists, triathletes, and martial artists:

- Bootcamp workouts—outdoors and indoors

- CrossFit workouts

- High-intensity interval training

- Leg, arm, and core workouts

All exercises can apply to the beginner or advanced fitness enthusiast, even if he does not participate in that particular sport. The circuit training examples at the ends of each section will help to create a training plan based on fitness level.

Strength training does not have to be complicated or expensive. The great thing about strength and stability training is that there are countless exercises that can be done without expensive equipment. For each exercise, you will see a star by the exercise title, noting the difficulty level of that exercise:

Beginner   ★

Advanced   ★ ★

Experienced   ★ ★ ★

# 3.1 RUNNERS

Following are nine strength and stability exercises for runners.

### Exercise 1: Push-Up ★ ★ ★

Muscles trained: back—chest—arms

Equipment: Exercise band

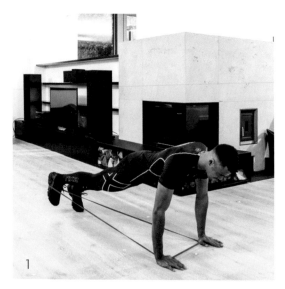 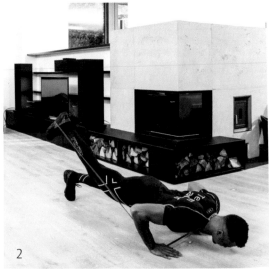

Procedure: Start in a prone position with hands placed shoulder-width apart and feet placed approximately hip-width apart. Keep the head aligned with the spine and maintain a straight body position. Place the light resistance band between the thumb and hand as well as unilaterally (i.e., one leg) under the foot. Keep the leg with the exercise band under the foot elevated at all times as you perform your push-ups. Flex your arms at least 90 degrees, lowering the body, and then return to original position with arms fully extended and leg raised. Repeat for the desired number of repetitions.

NOTE: Avoid driving the chin toward the chest or allowing the hips to sag. Keep a steady pace during both the concentric and eccentric phases.

# Exercise 2: CLX Side Plank ★

Muscles trained: shoulders—back—obliques

Equipment: TheraBand CLX

Procedure: Start in lateral plank position with your left forearm arm and side of the left foot on the floor. No other part of the body should be touching the floor. Place the TheraBand CLX over the foot so that it does not slip off. Hold the CLX band in the right hand. Straighten the right arm so it is pointed laterally. Rotate the arm with CLX band horizontally to chest level, then continue reaching with the arm until it is between the floor and left side of the torso. Then return to the starting position and repeat. Maintain a rigid core throughout the movement. Once you have completed all the repetitions on one side, repeat the exercise on the other side.

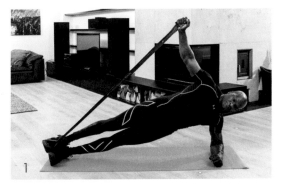

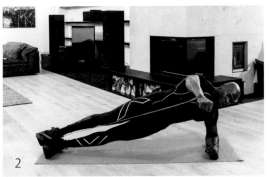

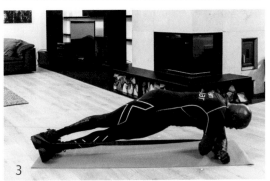

### Exercise 3:  Mountain Climber With a Chair ★

Muscles trained: shoulders—chest—back—abs—hips

Equipment: Chair

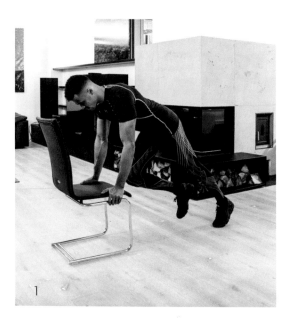 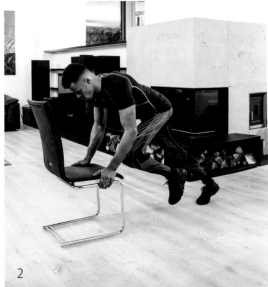

Procedure: Get into pronated position in front of the chair with your both of your hands shoulder-width apart on the sides of the chair. In this position, your upper body is elevated higher than your feet, making the exercise easier to perform. Stabilize your torso and keep your head and neck straight and aligned with your spine. Proceed to dynamically bring your knees into your chest, alternating legs. This will resemble running in place. Repeat for the desired number of repetitions.

## Exercise 4:  Foam Roller Passive Push-Up With Knee Flexion ★★

Muscles trained: arms—hips—chest—back

Equipment: Foam roller

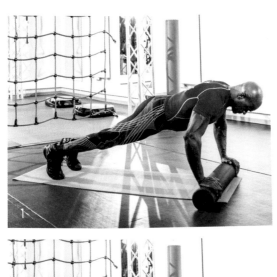

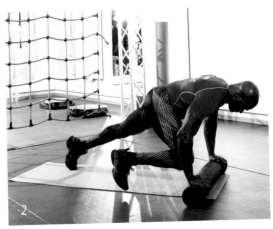

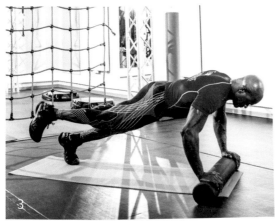

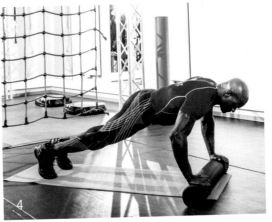

Procedure: Start from a push-up position with both hands on the foam roller at shoulder width. Then perform a push-up by flexing and extending your elbows. Bring one knee into the chest and then extend the leg behind you. Alternate legs with each push-up. It is important to hold the leg in the eccentric position for about 5 seconds before switching legs. Repeat for the desired number of repetitions.

## Exercise 5:   Lying Foam Roller Crossover ★ ★

Muscles trained: abs—lower back

Equipment: Foam roller

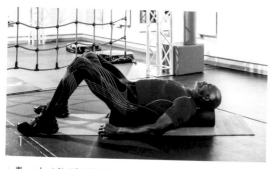

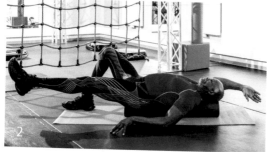

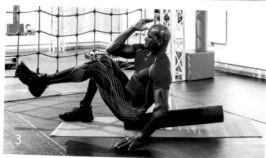

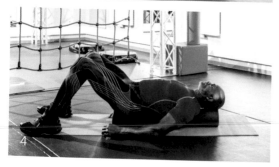

Procedure: Lie down with your vertebrae column on the foam roller, making sure that neck and head are secure. Place the left arm down by your side and the right arm slightly beside your ear. Keeping your back flat on the foam roller, extend your left leg at the knee and raise your heel away from the floor. Your right leg is flexed at the knee with the foot on the floor. Then contralaterally curl and twist your torso, keeping the chin tilted upward and the left hand on the floor. With a slight swing, cross your right elbow contralaterally to the left knee. Return to the starting position and then repeat. Make sure to complete the same number of repetitions on both sides.

## Exercise 6: Foam Roller Jackknife (Balance) ★

Muscles trained: abs—lower back

Equipment: Foam roller

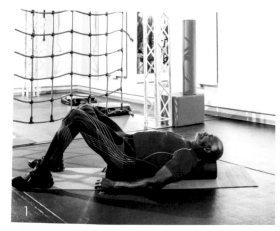

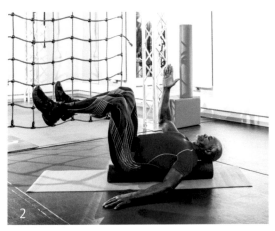

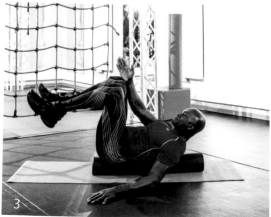

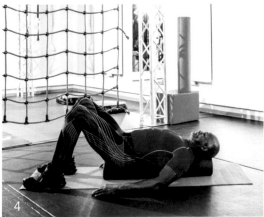

Procedure: Lie down with your vertebrae column on the foam roller, making sure the neck and head are secure. Place the left arm down by your side and the right arm slightly beside your head. With your back flat on the foam roller, raise both of your legs, bending at the knees, and lift your heels away from the floor. Then, like a jackknife, curl your knees, bringing them to your torso. Keep the chin tilted up. The left hand stays on the floor, and with a slight swing, move the right arm along the right side of the torso in the sagittal plane beside the right knee. Return to the starting position and then repeat. After you complete all repetitions on one side, repeat the exercise on the other side.

## Exercise 7:   Exercise Band Hyperextension ★

Muscles trained: back—arms

Equipment: Exercise band, exercise mat

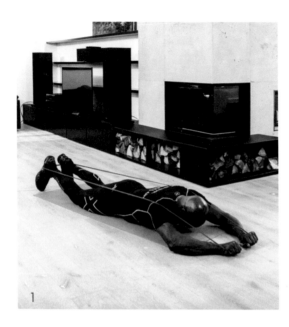 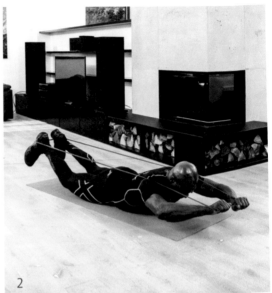

Procedure: Lie on the mat in a pronated position (on your stomach). Hold the light resistance band in both of your hands with your arms stretched out in front of you. The band should also be under both of your feet with your legs stretched out. The band is dorsal positioned, meaning behind the body when in the facedown position. Then lift arms and legs off the floor at the same time. Return to the starting position and repeat.

## Exercise 8:  Bodyweight Squat With a Chair  ★

Muscles trained: legs—hips

Equipment: Chair

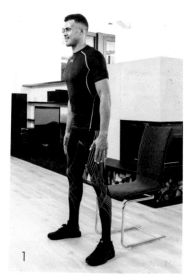 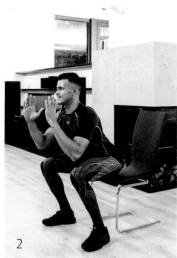 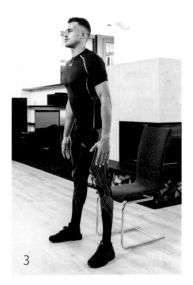

Procedure: Position in front of the chair with your back to the chair and your heels about 5 to 8 inches away. With your arms at your side, proceed to perform a 90-degree bodyweight squat, stopping when your buttocks lightly touch the chair. Do not sit down but rather slightly tap the chair with your buttocks. While you are performing the squat, raise your arms in front of you, abducting them about 60 degrees in the sagittal plane, and adduct them (lower the arms) as you stand back up straight. Then repeat the exercise.

## Exercise 9:   Backward to Forward Lunge With 90-Degree Elbow Bend ★

Muscles trained: arms—legs—back

Equipment: Gymstick Aerobic Bar

Procedure: Stand with aerobic bar in the second lever arm position—arm is flexed with the elbow at 90 degrees. Then perform a forward lunge. Bring the back leg up, and then immediately step back into a backward lunge. Stand back up straight, and then start the forward lunge with the opposite leg. Repeat the exercise.

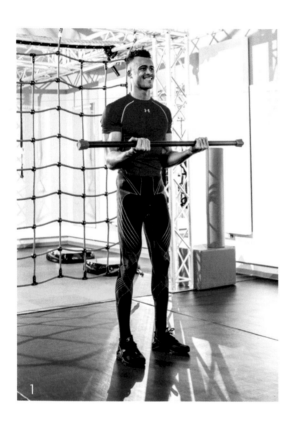

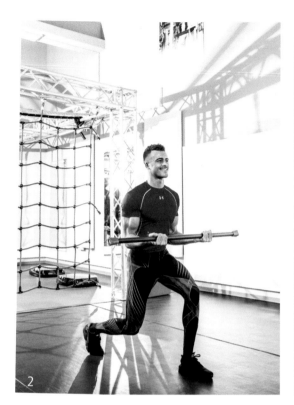

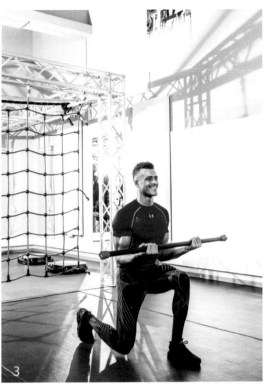

Using the previous nine exercises, perform circuit training two to three times a week for 20 to 30 minutes. There are two circuit variations, one for beginners and another for advanced exercisers (see the following tables). The breaks between exercises, unless otherwise specified, should last only as long as needed to change position. This will ensure that the circuit training is effective.

## Circuit Training for Beginners

| EXERCISE | SETS AND REPS | REST (SECONDS) |
|---|---|---|
| 1 Push-Up | 15x | — |
| 5 Lying Foam Roller Crossover | 2 x 10 | 15 |
| 6 Foam Roller Jackknife (Balance) | 10x per side | — |
| 3 Mountain Climber With a Chair | 3 x 15 seconds | 15 |
| 7 Exercise Band Hyperextension | 2 x 10 | 15 |
| 2 CLX Side Plank | 2x per side, hold for 15 seconds | — |
| 8 Bodyweight Squat With a Chair | 10x | — |
| 9 Backward to Forward Lunge With 90-Degree Elbow Bend | 10x per leg | — |
| NOTE: Take a one- to two-minute break, and then repeat all exercises. | | |

Running alone is not enough, especially for people who work in an office. Sitting for several hours a day leads to muscular imbalances. Even when walking, some muscle groups become stronger while other muscles are shortened or even become weaker, leading also to muscular imbalance. To prevent this, we have the nine most important balancing exercises for runners. You only need to do the exercises three times a week—so no excuses! Here we go.

## Advanced Circuit Training

| EXERCISE | SETS AND REPS | REST (SECONDS) |
|---|---|---|
| 1 Push-Up | 15-20x | — |
| 5 Lying Foam Roller Crossover | 2 x 25 | 15 |
| 6 Foam Roller Jackknife (Balance) | 15x per side | — |
| 3 Mountain Climber With a Chair | 2 x 30 seconds | 10 |
| 7 Exercise Band Hyperextension | 2 x 20 | 10 |
| 2 CLX Side Plank | 3x per side, hold for 25 secondsw | — |
| 8 Bodyweight Squat With a Chair | 15-20x | — |
| 9 Backward to Forward Lunge With 90-Degree Elbow Bend | 15x per leg | — |
| NOTE: Take a one- to two-minute break, and then repeat all exercises. | | |

# 3.2 CYCLISTS

Following are nine strength and stability exercises for cyclists.

### Exercise 1:   Medicine Ball Walkover ★ ★

Muscles trained: arms–chest–back–abs

Equipment: Medicine ball, pillow

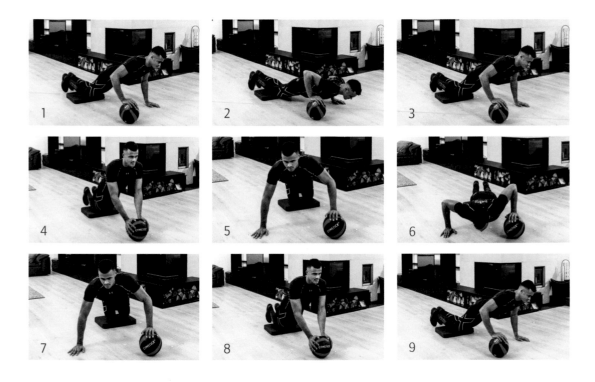

Procedure: With the medicine ball under your chest, put your right hand on the ball. Place your knees on a pillow or cushion. Keeping your core tight, start inhaling and lower your body as far as you can. Pause at the bottom and then push back up to the starting position while exhaling. Do not drop your hips! Your head should stay in the same position from start to finish. Then switch by putting the left hand on the ball together with the right hand, and then move the right hand to the floor under the shoulder. Keeping your core tight, start inhaling and lower your body as far as you can. Pause at the bottom and then push back up to the starting position while exhaling. Then repeat exercise, starting again with the right hand on the medicine ball.

## Exercise 2:  Stability Ball Tap With Exercise Band  ★

Muscles trained: shoulders—back—hips

Equipment: Small stability ball, light resistance band

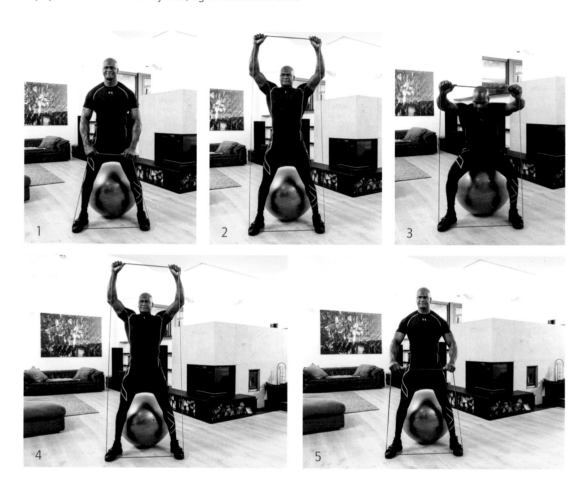

Procedure: Stand straight with feet apart directly in front of the stability ball. Position the exercise band under your feet. Hold the ends of the band in both hands, shoulder-width apart and at upper-thigh level. As you squat, raise your arms up, slightly touch the stability ball with your buttocks, and then stand back up, lowering your arms. Repeat the exercise.

## Exercise 3:  CLX Chest Press  ★

Muscles trained: arms—chest—shoulders

Equipment: TheraBand CLX

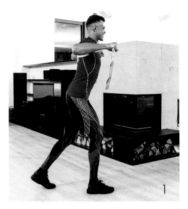
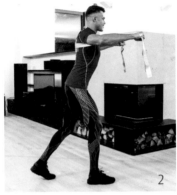
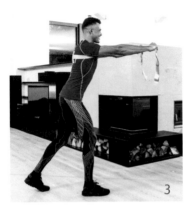
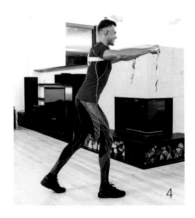
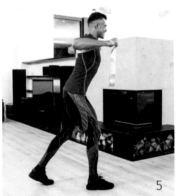

Procedure: Stand with your feet staggered. Bend both knees slightly. Place the CLX band behind your upper back. Hold the ends of the band in both hands, using the loops that best match your strength level, and extend in your arms in front of your body, keeping your elbows slightly bent. Press the band out in front of you, straightening your elbows. Bring your arms back in to the starting position. Repeat for the desired repetitions, and then switch legs so that the back leg is in front, and repeat.

# Exercise 4: CLX Diagonal Chop ★

Muscles trained: abs—back

Equipment: TheraBand CLX

Procedure: For this exercise, you can use a partner. If you do not have a partner, you must have the proper door or window anchor equipment. If you have a partner, the partner that is assisting by holding the CLX band should have the CLX held as low as possible. Then you should take CLX band and find the loop that is best for your strength level. Turn 90 degrees away from your partner or anchor position. Stand with the feet wide apart and raise the heel of the foot nearest the CLX band. Place the far hand over the other hand or interlace fingers.

Keeping your arms straight, pull CLX band diagonally upward around the shoulders by rotating torso, bending the knees, and raising the arms gradually up until the CLX band contacts the body. Return to the starting position and repeat on the opposite side.

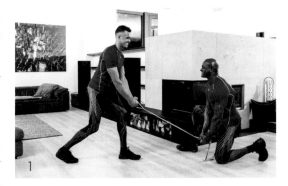

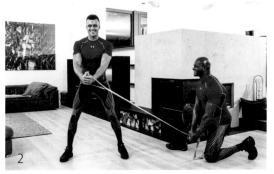

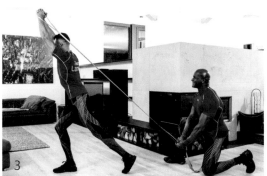

## Exercise 5:  CLX Lateral Glute Abduction ★

Muscles trained: hips

Equipment: TheraBand CLX

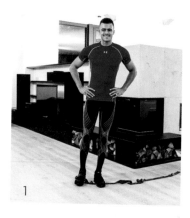
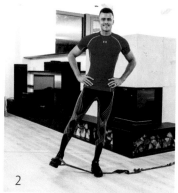
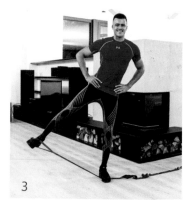
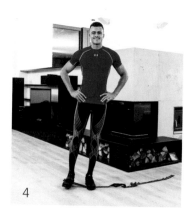
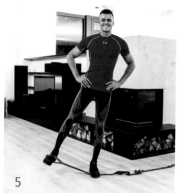
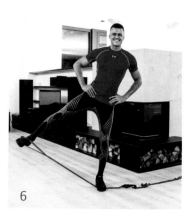

Procedure: Stand with the left foot on the CLX band. This way you can provide resistance for the right leg. Then place your right foot in the correct loop depending on the resistance you need. Place both hands on the hips, and then proceed to laterally abduct the leg away from your body. For stability, you must contract your stomach muscles and your back muscles. Finish the set on the right leg, and then switch and repeat on the left leg.

# Exercise 6:  CLX Hyperextension From the Glutes ★

Muscles trained: legs—hips

Equipment: TheraBand CLX

Procedure: Kneel down on your hands and knees. Keep hands shoulder-width apart and flat on the ground. You can place a pillow or cushion under your knees if needed for comfort and to keep your back straight. The CLX band should be held with the hand unilaterally on side of the leg and hip that you are training. Place your foot in the CLX loop for the best resistance that fits your training level. Then on the side you are training, lift the knee slightly from the floor and then extend the leg over the hip as for as you can. Return to the starting position. Repeat exercise on the other side.

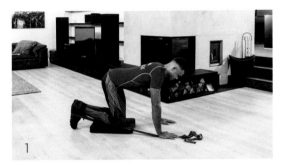

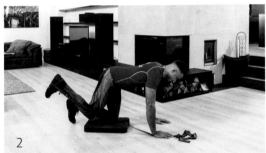

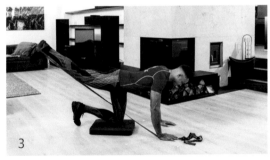

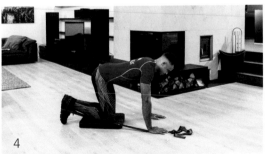

## Exercise 7:  Stability Ball Dead Bug ★ ★

Muscles trained: abs—oblques

Equipment: Stability ball

Procedure: Lying on your back, raise your legs and arms. Hold the stability ball between your toes and fingertips. Keeping your lower back on the floor, perform a contralateral movement of the arm–leg combination. Contralateral is always left arm and right leg and then switch to right arm and left leg. Continue contralaterally moving arms and legs for the required repetitions.

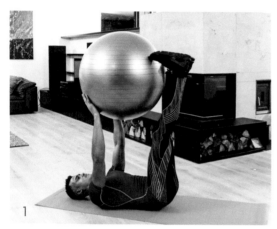
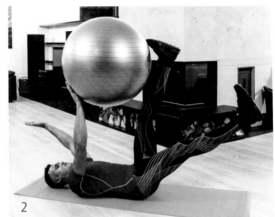
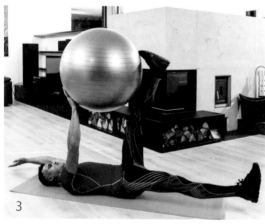
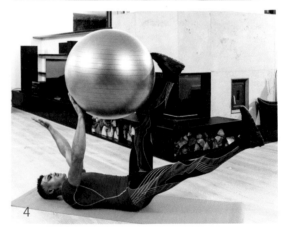

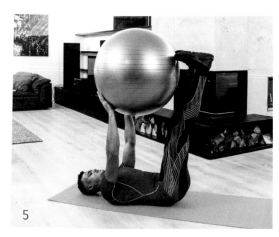

5

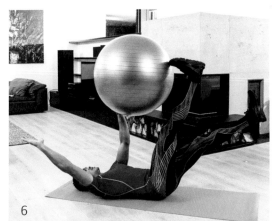

6

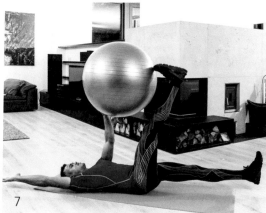

7

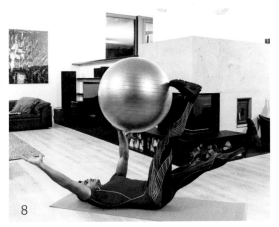

8

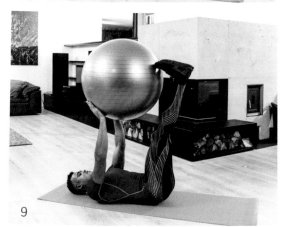

9

## Exercise 8: CLX Shoulder Press ★ ★

Muscles trained: arms—shoulders

Equipment: TheraBand CLX

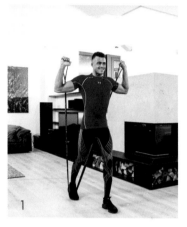
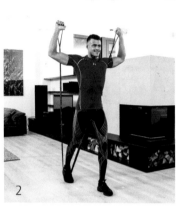
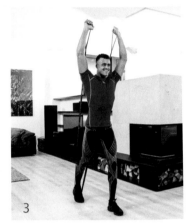

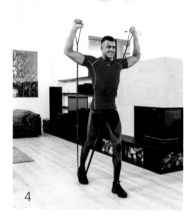
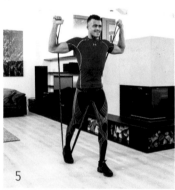

Procedure: Stagger your feet, placing the CLX band under the middle of your back foot. Position your hands inside the small loop holes for your resistance level. Then raise your arms laterally, keeping the elbows bent at 90 degrees. Press the CLX band up and out over your head, extending the elbows. Lean slightly into the resistance of the CLX band so that the resistance is slightly behind your head. Make sure to contract your lats, buttocks, and abs for added stability. After the set is complete, stagger the legs again by moving the back leg in front and the front leg in back, and then repeat the exercise.

# Exercise 9: CLX Seated Hamstring ★

Muscles trained: legs

Equipment: TheraBand CLX, chair

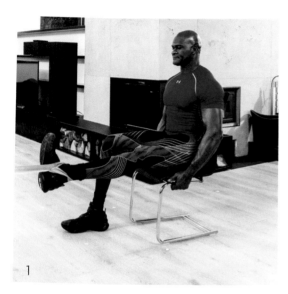 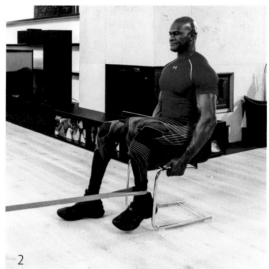

Procedure: This exercise is best performed sitting on a chair or on a massage table or something similar. Make sure the band is securely tied or held by a training partner before starting the exercise. Extend one knee, raising the leg until it is parallel to the floor. Ensure that you allow the knee to move to this extended position slowly and with control. Always sit upright and keep stable by holding on or by contracting your muscles. Pull band attachment back by flexing the knee until the knee is fully flexed, returning to the starting position. Repeat.

Using the nine exercises presented here, complete circuit training two to three times a week for 20 to 30 minutes. There are two different circuits, one for beginners and another for advanced exercisers. Each circuit takes about 20 to 30 minutes. The breaks between exercises, unless otherwise specified, should only last as long as it takes you to change position. This will make the circuit training more effective.

## Circuit Training for Beginners

| EXERCISE | SETS AND REPS | REST (SECONDS) |
| --- | --- | --- |
| 1 Medicine Ball Walkover | 5 x 10-15 | — |
| 2 Stability Ball Tap With Exercise Band | 3 x 20 | 15 |
| 3 CLX Chest Press | 4 x 15 | 10 |
| 4 CLX Diagonal Chop | 2 x 4 x 20 | 10 |
| 5 CLX Lateral Glute Abduction | 2x per side, hold for 25 seconds | — |
| 7 Stability Ball Dead Bug | 2 x 30 | — |
| 8 CLX Shoulder Press | 3 x 20 | — |
| 9 CLX Seated Hamstring | 4 x 15 per leg | — |
| NOTE: Take a one- to two-minute break, and then repeat the exercises. | | |

Cycling alone is not enough, especially for people who work in an office. Sitting for several hours a day leads to muscular imbalances. When cycling, some muscle groups become stronger while other muscles are shortened or even become weaker, leading also to muscular imbalance. To prevent this, we have the nine most important balancing exercises for cyclists. You only need to do the exercises three times a week—so no excuses! Here we go.

## Advanced Circuit Training

| EXERCISE | SETS AND REPS | REST (SECONDS) |
|---|---|---|
| 1 Medicine Ball Walkover | 5 x 15-20 | – |
| 2 Stability Ball Tap With Exercise Band | 3 x 25 | 15 |
| 3 CLX Chest Press | 4 x 25 | 10 |
| 4 CLX Diagonal Chop | 4 x 4 x 20 | 10 |
| 5 CLX Lateral Glute Abduction | Hold 4 x leg for 25 seconds | – |
| 7 Stability Ball Dead Bug | 4 x 30 | – |
| 8 CLX Shoulder Press | 3 x 25 | – |
| 9 CLX Seated Hamstring | 4 x 25 per leg | – |
| NOTE: Take a one- to two-minute break, and then repeat the exercises. | | |

# 3.3 TRIATHLETES

Following are nine strength and stability exercises for triathletes.

### Exercise 1:  Exercise Band Diagonal Rotation ★

Muscles trained: abs—hips—back

Equipment: Light resistance band

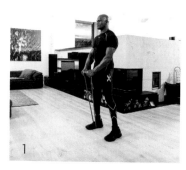
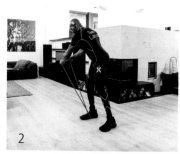
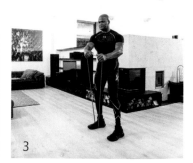
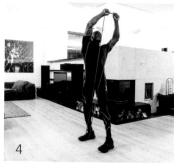
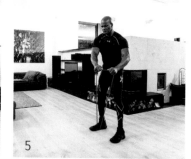
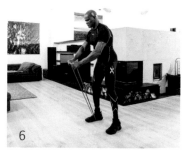

Procedure: First place the exercise band under the right foot. Stand up straight but in a slightly dynamic starting position, meaning knees are slightly bent, hips are pushed back slightly, and the arms are straight with the elbows bent at about 50 degrees. Rotate to the right about 20 degrees, keeping the arms next to the body. Make sure that there is enough resistance on the bands between the feet and the hands at all times to keep the muscles contracted. Now start to rotate diagonally to the left until your arms are above your head over your left shoulder. Keep the arms straight (with soft elbows) throughout. Hold the ending position, hyperextending slightly over the bent knees but not over the lower back. Hold for two seconds. Return to the starting position and repeat. After the desired repetitions, repeat the exercise on the opposite side with the exercise band under the left foot.

# Exercise 2: Exercise Band Abduction and Adduction With Side Step ★

Muscles trained: hips—legs

Equipment: Light resistance band

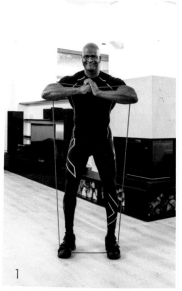
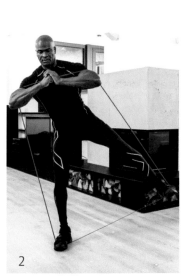
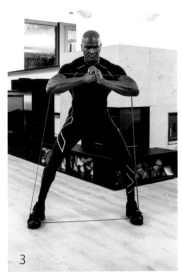

Procedure: To start, place the exercise band under the middle of the feet. It should be laterally positioned on both sides of the body, coming up to about midway of the upper arm. The arms are flexed at the elbow and abducted out of the shoulder joint to about 80 degrees to support the exercise band. Then, abduct the left leg as far as possible. Because of the resistance band, the leg will adduct immediately. So be sure to take a wide sumo-type step and slightly squat about 40 degrees or deeper, if desired. Return to starting position and repeat.

## Exercise 3:  Exercise Band Rotation ★

Muscles trained: shoulders—arms—back

Equipment: Light resistance band

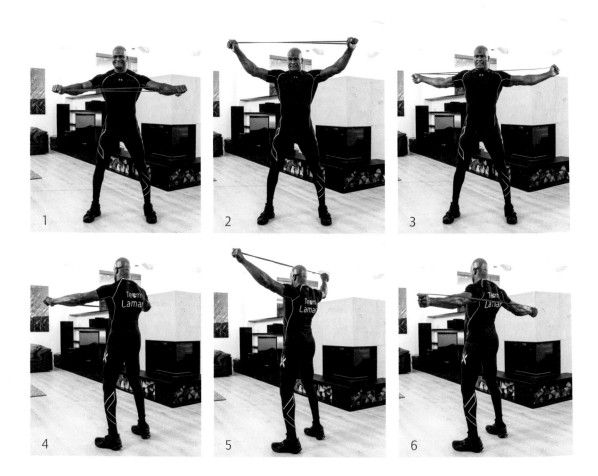

Procedure: Start with feet shoulder-width apart and the exercise band in both hands. Position arms laterally and parallel to the floor at chest level. Then, with both arms slightly over the shoulder joint, begin to laterally rotate over the shoulder joint into hyperextension until you feel the scapular muscles as well as the rhomboids. Return to the starting position and repeat.

# Exercise 4: Push-Up on Foam Roller ★ ★

Muscles trained: chest—arms—shoulders

Equipment: Foam roller, mat, Gymstick Aerobic Bar

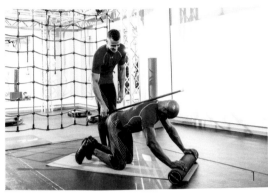
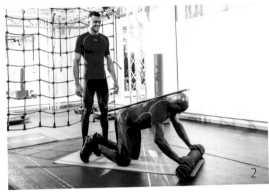
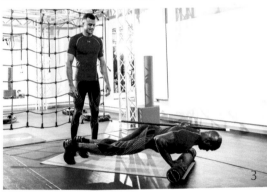
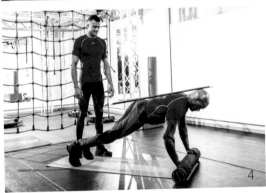

Procedure: Kneel on the floor and put both hands on the foam roller. You can have a partner place a Gymstick on your back aligned with your spine. The stick should be straight from your head to your hips. Lower into a push-up, and then extend the elbows, rising to the starting position. The Gymstick should remain in line with your spine from your head to your hips throughout the entire exercise. Repeat for the desired repetitions.

## Exercise 5: CLX Side Plank Abduction With Rotation ★ ★ ★

Muscles trained: back—obliques—shoulders

Equipment: TheraBand CLX, exercise mat

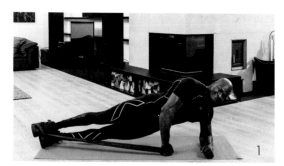

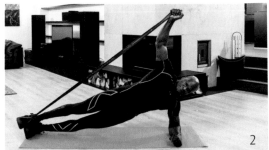

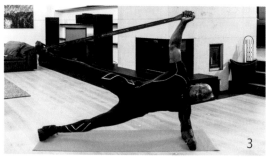

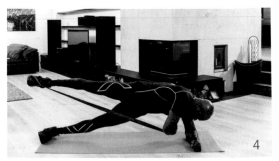

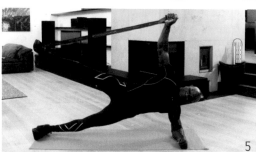

Procedure: Start in the side plank position with left forearm arm and side of left foot on the ground. No other part of the body should be touching the floor. Place the CLX band over the foot so it does not slip off. Also hold the CLX band in the right hand. The right arm is straight and pointed laterally out of the shoulder joint. Then, lift the right leg laterally. Keeping the leg contracted and open, rotate the right arm horizontally at chest level. Continue rotating the arm until it is between the floor and left side of the torso. Return to the starting position and repeat for desired repetitions. Then complete the exercise on the opposite side.

# Exercise 6:  Exercise Band Core Hyperextension ★

Muscles trained: back

Equipment: Light resistance band, exercise mat

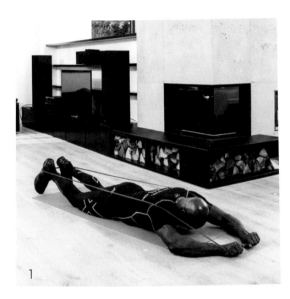 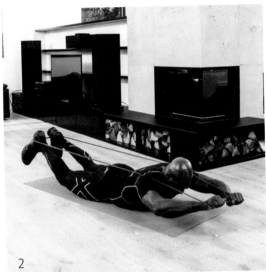

Procedure: Lie on your stomach in the pronated position. Hold the exercise band in both hands with arms stretched out in front of you. The band should also be anchored under both of your feet and your legs stretched out behind you. The band is positioned behind the back of the body when in the facedown position. Then lift arms and legs off the floor at the same time. Return to the starting position and repeat.

## Exercise 7: Stability Ball Lateral Reach ★ ★

Muscles trained: back—shoulders

Equipment: Stability ball, light resistance band

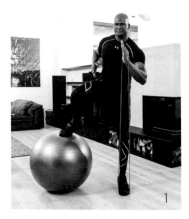 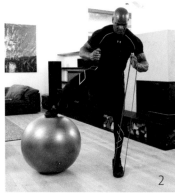 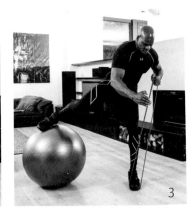

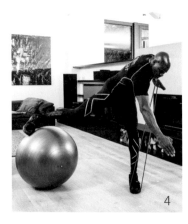 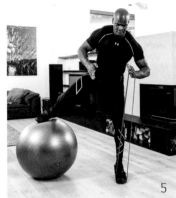 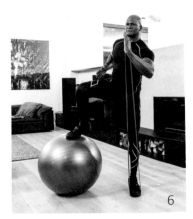

Procedure: Place the toes of your right foot on the stability ball. Position the exercise band under your left foot and hold it in your left hand. The exercise band should be held between the thumb and pointer finger, and all fingers should be extended straight. Then perform a lateral lunge on the stability ball while at the same time rotating to the left. Increase the resistance by reaching with the right hand. Return to the starting position while still using the exercise band to keep resistance on the left arm and torso as you slightly rotate and abduct the upper arm away from the torso. After desired repetitions, repeat on the opposite side.

## Exercise 8:  Medicine Ball One-Arm Push-Up ★ ★ ★

Muscles trained: abs—back—shoulders—chest

Equipment: Medicine ball

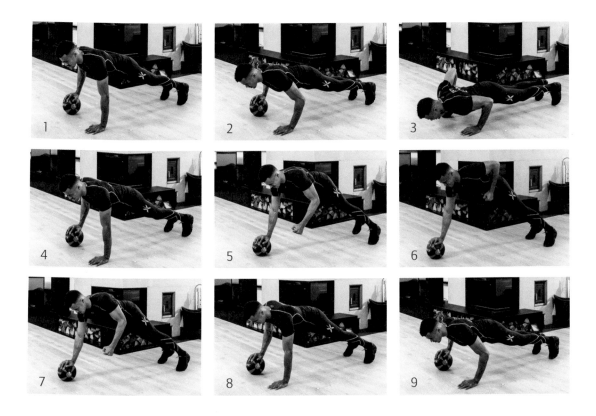

Procedure: With the medicine ball directly under your chest, place your right hand on the ball. Keeping your core tight, inhale and lower your body as far as you can. Pause at the bottom and then push back up to the starting position while exhaling. Do not drop your hips! Your head should stay in the same position from start to finish. Then lift the left arm from extension to hyperextension as far as you can and hold for 2 or 3 seconds, keeping your core tight. Then return to the starting position with left hand on the floor and repeat the exercise.

NOTE: This exercise is very advanced, so only attempt once you have mastered the basic push-up with one hand on a medicine ball.

## Exercise 9:   Jump Rope High Step  ★ ★ ★

Muscles trained: legs–shoulders–back–arms–chest

Lower body: Though the calves are the main muscles powering the jump, your quadriceps, hamstrings, and glutes are also activated. The load phase of rolling through the ball of your foot and pushing off with the toes calls the posterior side of your body, the glutes, hamstrings, and calves, into action. The quadriceps and glutes then help you to control the jump and land lightly on your feet rather than hitting the floor with a thud. The knees should be slightly bent during both the push-off and landing phases of the jump.

Upper body: The shoulders and abs are the upper-body power muscles when jumping rope, though the arms and hands also help to swing the rope. Your back along with your core stabilize your upper body, which should be elongated, straight, and centered over your pelvis rather than leaning forward or backward.

Equipment: Jump rope

Procedure: Traditionally, jumping rope falls under cardiovascular exercise. When jump ropes are used for longer duration sessions, you can burn a lot calories. The great thing about varying your jump rope training to include shorter, high-intensity interval sets (especially with a weighted rope) is that you are getting much higher muscle activation and recruiting more muscle fibers for both upper and lower body. This will help you build muscle over time, which can make your body more efficient at burning calories. Think of the difference between a distance runner's physique and a sprinter's physique and that will give you a good analogy of the different results you can get from varied jump rope training routines. They are very portable. If you are traveling or have limited space in your gym bag, it's a convenient tool to have. The initial difficulty of learning to jump is often a barrier for people. It takes time and effort to learn to jump rope and learn a variety of skills, and that's why you might not see a whole lot of individuals jumping at the gym. Anyone can hop on a machine. Learning to jump is a very satisfying feeling. It keeps people engaged and challenged and helps to avoid the monotony inherent in many other types of cardiovascular exercises that lead to disinterest. You can get a decent jump rope for a few bucks. Depending on your fitness level, jump rope for approximately one to two minutes without stopping.

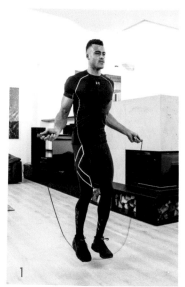

1

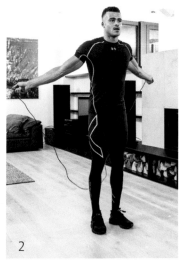

2

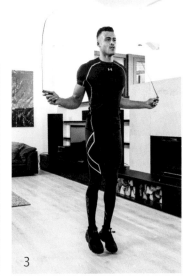

3

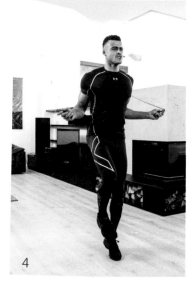

4

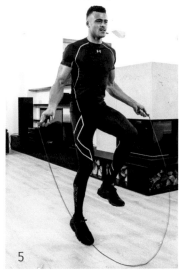

5

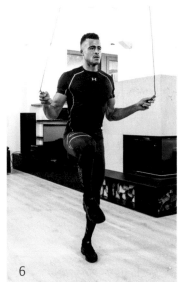

6

# FUNCTIONAL FITNESS AT HOME

Using the previous nine exercises, perform circuit training two to three times a week for 20 to 30 minutes. There are two circuit variations, one for beginners and another for advanced exercisers (see the following tables). The breaks between exercises, unless otherwise specified, should last only as long as needed to change position. This will ensure that the circuit training is effective.

## Circuit Training for Beginners

| EXERCISE | SETS AND REPS | REST (SECONDS) |
|---|---|---|
| 1 Exercise Band Diagonal Rotation | 2 x 15 each side | — |
| 2 Exercise Band Abduction and Adduction With Side Step | 3 x 15 | 30 |
| 3 Exercise Band Rotation | 3 x 20 each side | — |
| 4 Push-Up on Foam Roller | 3 x 20 each side | — |
| 5 CLX Side Plank Abduction With Rotation | 3 x 20 each side | — |
| 6 Exercise Band Core Hyperextension | 5 x 20 | — |
| 7 Stability Ball Lateral Reach | 4 x 20 | — |
| 8 Medicine Ball One-Arm Push-Up | 3 x 15 each arm | — |
| 9 Jump Rope High Step | 3 x 1:30 minutes | — |
| NOTE: Take a one- to two-minute break, and then repeat all exercises. | | |

The nine exercises presented in this chapter are meant to strengthen the trunk muscles, legs, and arms. These exercises can all be done at home. Strength training is required for every sport, but most still neglect it. During a sport season, these exercises should be performed twice a week; they should be performed three times a week during the off-season. A professional trainer can also advise how often you should perform the exercises as part of your training.

## Advanced Circuit Training

| EXERCISE | SETS AND REPS | REST |
|---|---|---|
| 1 Exercise Band Diagonal Rotation | 4 x 25 each side | — |
| 2 Exercise Band Abduction and Adduction With Side Step | 4 x 25 each side | 15 |
| 3 Exercise Band Rotation | 4 x 25 each side | — |
| 4 Push-Up on Foam Roller | 4 x 25 each side | — |
| 5 CLX Side Plank Abduction With Rotation | 4 x 30 each side | 10 |
| 6 Exercise Band Core Hyperextension | 5 x 30 | 10 |
| 7 Stability Ball Lateral Reach | Hold 30x each side for 25 seconds | — |
| 9 Jump Rope High Step | 4 x 2 minutes | — |
| NOTE: Take a one- to two-minute break, and then repeat all exercises. | | |

# 3.4 MARTIAL ARTS

Following are eight strength and stability exercises for martial artists.

### Exercise 1:  CLX Chest Press 1  ★

Muscles trained: chest—arms

Equipment: TheraBand CLX

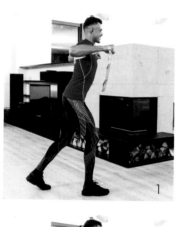
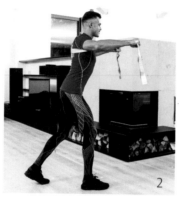
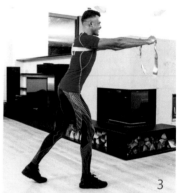
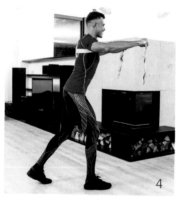
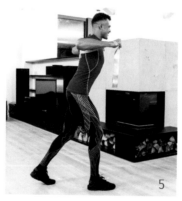

Procedure: Stand with your feet staggered and knees slightly bent. Place the CLX band behind your back at about shoulder blade height. Hold the loops that best fit your resistance level. Then position bands to the side of chest with elbows held high out to the sides. Forearms should be horizontal. Then lean into the resistance. Push the bands forward until your arms are extended and parallel to each other. Return to the stretching position until a slight stretch is felt in the chest or shoulders and repeat.

## Exercise 2:  CLX Chest Press 2 ★ ★

Muscles trained: chest—arms—shoulders—abs

Equipment: TheraBand CLX

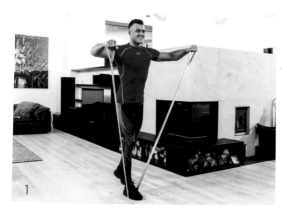

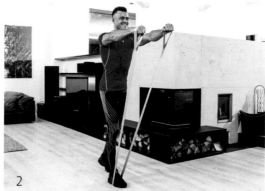

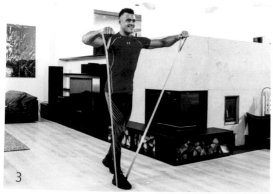

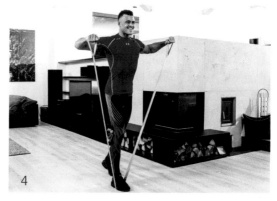

**Procedure:** Stand with your feet staggered and knees slightly bent. Place the CLX band under the leading foot. The band runs parallel from under your foot to your hands. Hold the loops that best match your resistance level. Because the bands are anchored below from your foot, the shoulder muscles will be very intensively involved is this exercise. Push the bands forward until your arms are extended and parallel to each other. Return to the stretching position until slight stretch is felt in the chest or shoulders and repeat.

## Exercise 3:  Core Hyperextension With Rotation ★ ★

Muscles trained: abs—back

Equipment: Stability ball, medicine ball

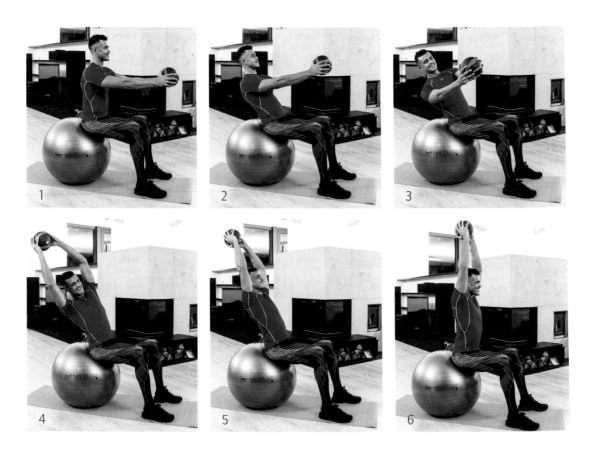

Procedure: When sitting on the stability ball for this exercise, it is important to remember to not sit centered on top of the ball but rather about 15 degrees down into the ball. Also, knees must be bent at 90 degrees with the feet shoulder-width apart. Throughout the exercise, keep the back straight, chest up, and chin parallel to the floor. Hold the medicine ball at chest level and straight out in front of you. The ball should not be too heavy. Then, hyperextend out of the hip joint by leaning slightly back, keeping the arms straight in front of the chest. Rotate to the right slightly, keeping the ball in front of the chest. Then, move the ball over your head, keeping your arms straight but still remaining in the hyperextended position. Flex your upper body back to the starting position. Then finally bring the arms back to a parallel position in front of your chest. Repeat exercise for the desired repetitions, and then repeat on the opposite side.

## Exercise 4: CLX Hip Flexor Hyperextension ★ ★

Muscles trained: legs

Equipment: TheraBand CLX

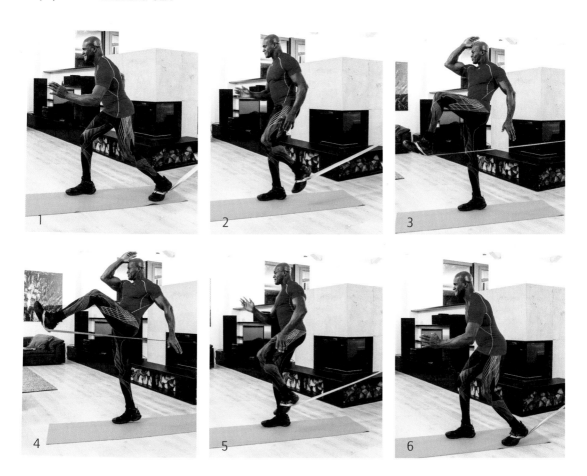

Procedure: Stand with your legs staggered. Loop the CLX band behind the back foot. Either have the band anchored low or held low by a partner. Begin to hyperextend the hip flexor by bring your back leg up so that the thigh is parallel to the floor. Keep the knee flexed throughout. Bring your leg back to the starting position. Repeat for the desired repetitions, and then switch to the other leg. Activate your core stability and gluteal muscles to maintain good posture and a steady pelvis during the exercise. Do not lean your body to the side of the standing leg. Swing your arms reciprocally with your leg as you carry out the sprinting motion.

## Exercise 5:  Unilateral Push-Up  ★ ★ ★

Muscles trained: chest—back—shoulders—arms

Equipment: Hand towel

Procedure: Start with your hands and balls of your feet on the floor. Make sure the hands and feet are shoulder-width apart. Place small towels that are slightly folded under your hands. The towels provide an unstable environment for the chest as well as the spine, forcing you to recruit your core muscles for stability. Rotate the left arm 90 degrees from the shoulder joint, positioning the hand laterally. As the left arm slides sideways, abducting away from the torso, lower into a push-up. Extend back up by adducting the left arm and rotating the hand 90 degrees inward to the starting position. Repeat the exercise with right arm. Remember to keep the neck and head in alignment with the spine.

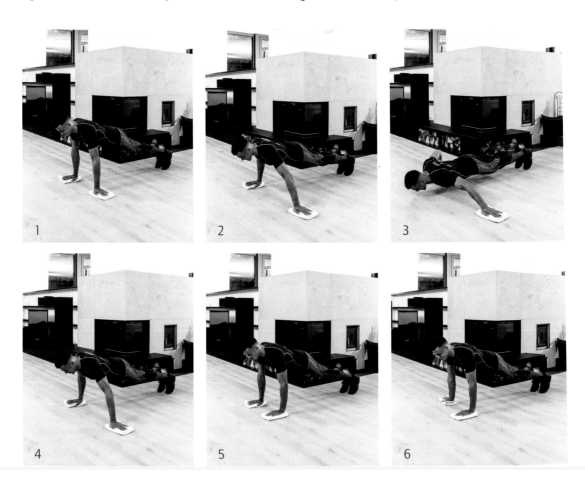

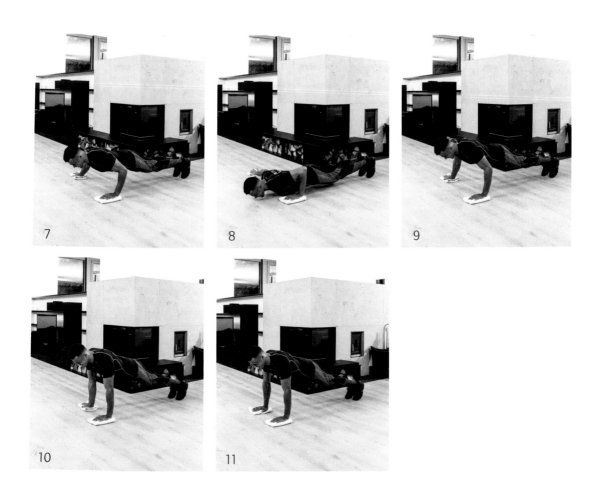

## Exercise 6:   Kettlebell Turkish Get-Up ★ ★ ★

Muscles trained: all muscle groups

Equipment: Kettlebell

Procedure: Lie flat on your back, holding a kettlebell in your right hand with your arm fully extended. Bend your right knee slightly, placing your right foot flat on the floor. While keeping the arm with the kettlebell extended throughout, use your free arm to help push yourself into a sitting position; then slowly progress to one knee. While keeping your balance and the kettlebell locked, slowly stand up. Return to the starting position and repeat movement for the desired repetitions, and then switch the kettlebell to the other hand.

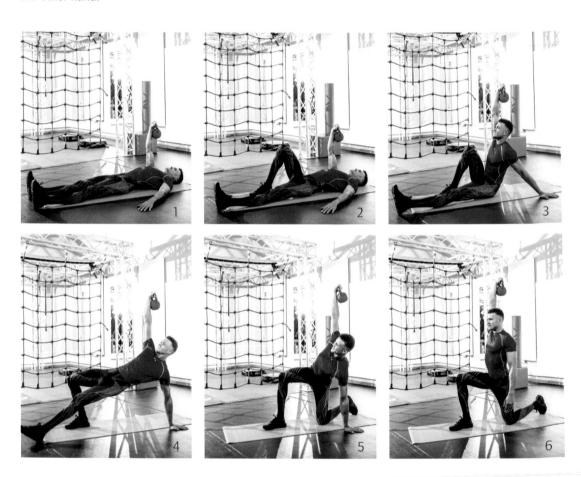

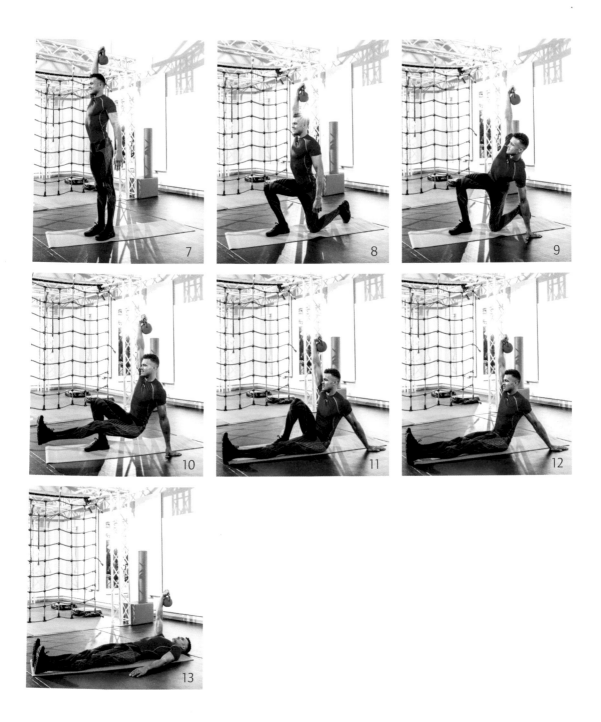

## Exercise 7: Kettlebell Double Swing With Jump ★ ★ ★

Muscles trained: all muscle groups

Equipment: Kettlebell

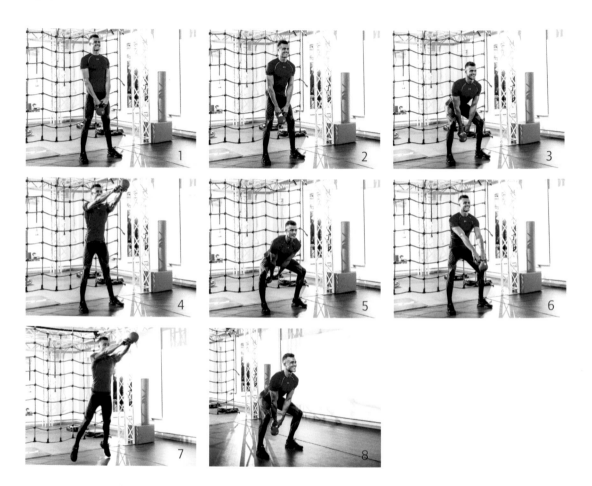

Procedure: Stand up straight with your feet placed shoulder-width apart. Bend your knees slightly and stick your butt out. Hold a kettlebell with both hands in an overhand grip. The kettlebell should be placed between your legs. Lift the kettlebell forward parallel to the chest and then let it fall back between your legs. Do this two times, and then on the third swing, take a plyometric jump forward as far as you can, making sure to bend at the knees as you land. Return to the starting position and repeat.

# Exercise 8: CLX Push With Contralateral Lunge ★ ★ ★

Muscles trained: chest–arms–shoulders

Equipment: TheraBand CLX

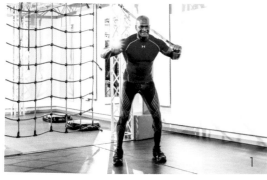
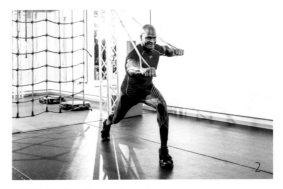
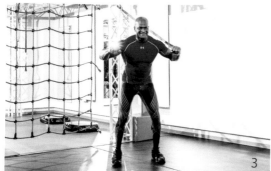
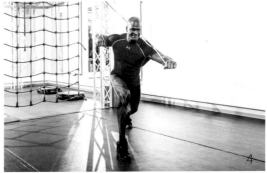

Procedure: Position the CLX band high behind the body. Stand with the legs and feet a bit wider than shoulder width. Take the CLX band from both sides and position the bands to the side of the chest with the elbows held high out to the sides. Forearms should be horizontal. Lean into the resistance and push the CLX band forward, alternating arms. Lunge forward at the same time until arms are extended. Return to the starting position until slight stretch is felt in chest or shoulders. CLX bands should follow a slight arc pattern as hands travel closer together toward extension.

## FUNCTIONAL FITNESS AT HOME

Using the previous eight exercises, perform circuit training two to three times a week for 20 to 30 minutes. There are two circuit variations, one for beginners and another for advanced exercisers (see the following tables). The breaks between exercises, unless otherwise specified, should last only as long as needed to change position. This will ensure that the circuit training is effective.

## Circuit Training for Beginners

| EXERCISE | SETS AND REPS | REST (SECONDS) |
|---|---|---|
| 1 CLX Chest Press 1 | 3 x 25 | – |
| 2 CLX Chest Press 2 | 3 x 20 | 10 |
| 3 Core Hyperextension With Rotation | 4 x 15 each side | – |
| 4 CLX Hip Flexor Hyperextension | 4 x 20 | – |
| 5 Unilateral Push-Up | 4 x 15 each side | – |
| 6 Kettlebell Turkish Get-Up | 3 x 15 each side | – |
| 7 Kettlebell Double Swing With Jump | 4 x 20 | – |
| 8 CLX Push With Contralateral Lunge | 4 x 15 each side | – |
| NOTE: Take a one- to two-minute break, and then repeat all the exercises. | | |

For all combat athletes, it is especially important to train for strength, endurance, load from top to bottom and vice versa, jumps, power kicks, as well as rotation with stability.

## Advanced Circuit Training

| EXERCISE | SETS AND REPS | REST (SECONDS) |
|---|---|---|
| 1 CLX Chest Press 1 | 4 x 25 | – |
| 2 CLX Chest Press 2 | 4 x 20 | 10 |
| 3 Core Hyperextension With Rotation | 5 x 15 each side | – |
| 4 CLX Hip Flexor Hyperextension | 4 x 25 | – |
| 5 Unilateral Push-Up | 4 x 20 each side | – |
| 6 Kettlebell Turkish Get-Up | 4 x 20 each side | – |
| 7 Kettlebell Double Swing With Jump | 4 x 30 | – |
| 8 CLX Push With Contralateral Lunge | 4 x 25 each side | – |
| NOTE: Take a one- to two-minute break, and then repeat all the exercises. | | |

# 3.5 BOOTCAMP WORKOUTS

These bootcamp workouts can be done indoors or outdoors.

### Exercise 1: Mountain Climber ★ ★

Muscles trained: all muscle groups

Equipment: None

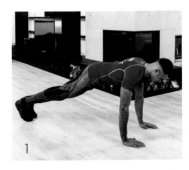 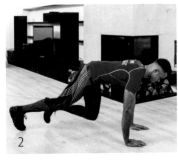 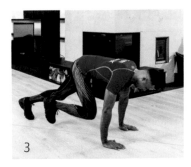

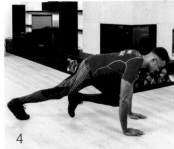 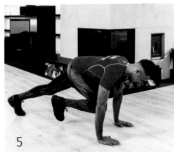

Procedure: Start in the push-up position. Hands are shoulder-width apart, and feet are hip-width apart. Keep the head aligned with the spine and maintain a straight body position throughout. Holding the push-up position, dynamically bring one knee into the chest. Fully extend the leg, returning to the starting position, and then bring the opposite knee into the chest. Alternate bringing the knees into the chest like you are running in place for the desired repetitions.

# Exercise 2: Burpee ★ ★ ★

Muscles trained: all muscle groups

Equipment: None

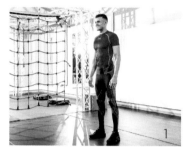
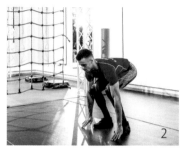
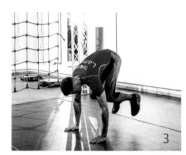

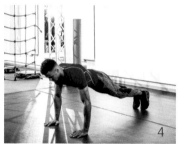
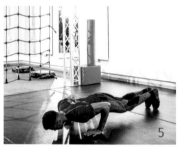
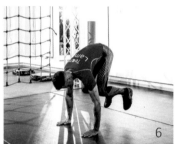

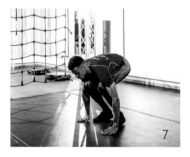

Procedure: Stand upright with the legs approximately hip-width apart and arms at the sides. Squat down to the crouched position, placing both hands on the floor. Immediately kick both legs back and assume a push-up position. Perform a bodyweight push-up. Next, reverse the movement back to the crouched position and immediately jump up vertically. Softly absorb the landing and stand upright with shoulders retracted. Keep the head aligned with the spine and the abdominals tight throughout the movement. Keep the legs parallel during each phase of the movement, and do not allow the hips to sag when extending from the crouched position. During the transition from the crouched position to the jump, allow the arms to naturally swing with the movement, providing additional momentum. Then repeat the entire series.

## Exercise 3:  CLX Side Plank With Upper-Body Rotation ★ ★ ★

Muscles trained: abs—obliques—back—shoulders

Equipment: TheraBand CLX

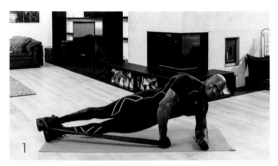

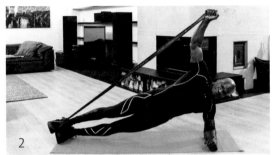

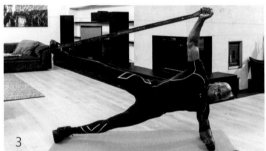

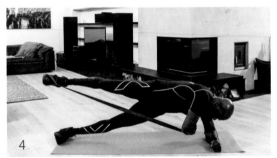

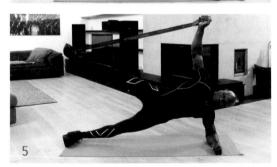

Procedure: Start in the side plank position with the left forearm and the side of the left foot on the floor. No other part of the body should be touching the floor. Place the CLX band over the foot so it does not slip off. Hold the CLX band in the right hand. The right arm is straight and pointed laterally out of the shoulder joint. Lift the right leg laterally and keep the leg contracted and open. Rotate the right arm horizontally at chest level, and then continue reaching until you go between the floor and left side of the body. Return to the starting position and repeat for the desired number of repetitions before switching to the other side.

## Exercise 4: Exercise Band Abduction With Side Step ★

Muscles trained: legs—hips

Equipment: Light resistance band

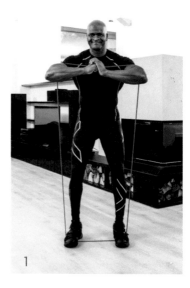 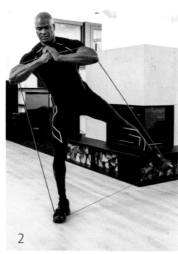 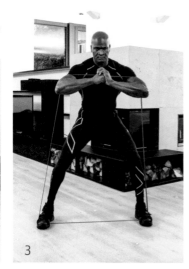

Procedure: Place the exercise band under the middle of the foot. It will be laterally positioned on both sides of the body, coming up to about midway of the upper arm. The elbows are flexed and abducted out of the shoulder joint to about 80 degrees to support the exercise band. Abduct the left leg as far as possible. The leg will adduct immediately because of the resistance from the band. Then take a sumo-type step and slightly squat about 40 degrees or deeper, if desired. Return to the starting position. After you complete the required repetitions on the left leg, repeat on the right leg.

## Exercise 5:  Medicine Ball Walkover  ★ ★ ★

Muscles trained: chest—shoulders—biceps—triceps—back

Equipment: Medicine ball

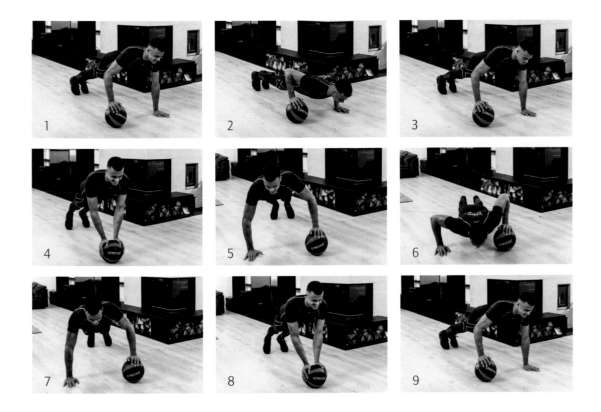

Procedure: Place the right hand on medicine ball, which should be directly under your chest. Keeping your core tight, inhale and lower your body as far as you can. Pause at the bottom and then push back up to the starting position while exhaling. Do not drop your hips! The head should stay in the same position from start to finish. Then switch by putting the left hand on the ball together with the right hand and then moving the right hand to the floor under the shoulder. Keeping your core tight, inhale and lower your body as far as you can. Pause at the bottom and then push back up to the starting position while exhaling. Do not drop your hips! Repeat exercise.

# Exercise 6: Diagonal Dorsal Loading ★ ★

Muscles trained: abs—shoulders—back

Equipment: Light resistance band

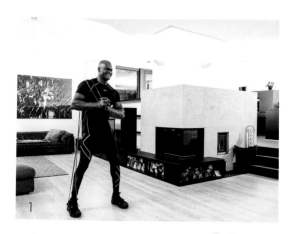

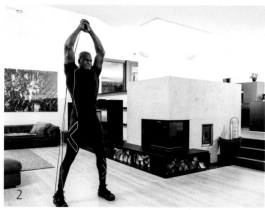

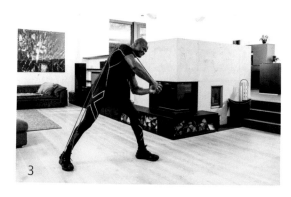

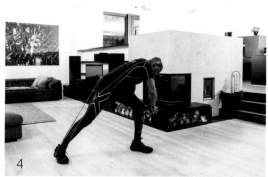

Procedure: Stand with the feet slightly sideways. Place the exercise band under your foot so that it runs behind your leg up to your hip, along your back to your shoulder, over the shoulder, and along the arm to your hand. The arms are abducted about 15 degrees from your body. This way you keep a large amount of resistance on the band, and it will not slide off the back or hip. Move your arms over your head and slightly rotate your torso in the direction of movement. Rotate diagonally down to the knee opposite the hand holding the band. Return to the starting position and repeat again for desired repetitions. Then complete exercise on the opposite side.

## Exercise 7:  CLX Shoulder Press ★ ★

Muscles trained: shoulders—arms

Equipment: TheraBand CLX

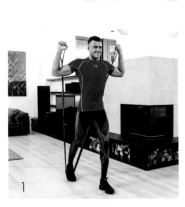 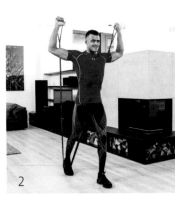 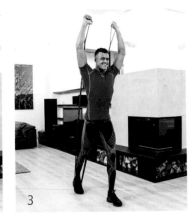

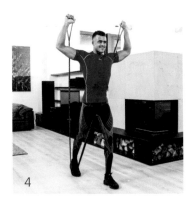 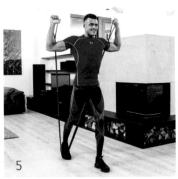

Procedure: Stagger your legs with one foot in front of the other. Place the CLX band under the middle of the back foot. Position your hands inside the small loops for your resistance level. Raise your arms laterally with the elbows bent at 90 degrees. Press the CLX band up and out in extension over your head. Lean slightly into the resistance of the CLX band so that the resistance is behind your head. Make sure to contract your lats, buttocks, and abs for added stability. Complete desired repetitions and then switch legs so opposite foot is in front, and repeat the exercise.

# Exercise 8: CLX Diagonal Chop ★ ★

Muscles trained: abs—back

Equipment: TheraBand CLX

Procedure: This exercise requires a partner. If you do not have a partner, then you must have the proper door or window anchor equipment. The partner holding the CLX band should have it held up as high as possible. Use the loop that is best for your strength category. Turn 90 degrees away from the partner or door. Position the feet wide apart and raise the heel of the foot nearest CLX band. Place the far hand over the other hand and interlace fingers.

Keeping arms straight, pull the CLX band diagonally down from above the left shoulder to below the right shoulder by rotating the torso and bending the knees. Keep the arms straight throughout. Return to the starting position and repeat on the opposite side. Continue for desired repetitions.

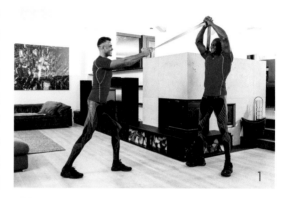

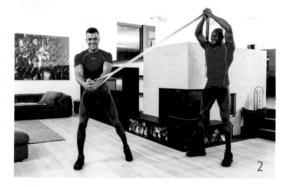

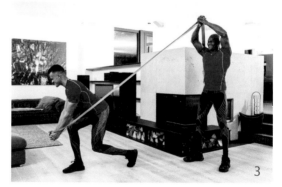

## FUNCTIONAL FITNESS AT HOME

Using the previous eight exercises, perform circuit training two to three times a week for 20 to 30 minutes. There are two circuit variations, with circuit II being slightly more advanced than circuit I (see the following tables). The breaks between exercises, unless otherwise specified, should last only as long as needed to change position. This will ensure that the circuit training is effective.

## Circuit Training I

| EXERCISE | SETS AND REPS | REST (SECONDS) |
|---|---|---|
| 1 Mountain Climber | 30 sec. | 30 |
| 7 CLX Shoulder Press | 15x | 30 |
| 8 CLX Diagonal Chop | 10 x each side | 30 |
| 2 Burpee | 30 sec. | 30 |
| 6 Diagonal Dorsal Loading | 10x | 30 |
| 5 Medicine Ball Walkover | 10 x side to side | 30 |
| 4 Exercise Band Abduction With Side Step | 10 x each side | 30 |
| 3 CLX Side Plank With Upper-Body Rotation | 10 x each side | 30 |
| NOTE: Take a one- to two-minute break, and then repeat all the exercises. | | |

Bootcamp training can be short and effective when done using these eight exercises. It is a high-intensity workout, giving you the maximum amount of benefits in the shortest amount of time. Generally, bootcamp workouts are designed as functional circuit training that can be done alone or in a small group.

## Circuit Training II

| EXERCISE | SETS AND REPS | REST (SECONDS) |
|---|---|---|
| 1 Mountain Climber | 45 sec. | 15 |
| 2 Burpee | 45 sec. | 15 |
| 7 CLX Shoulder Press | 20x | 15 |
| 8 CLX Diagonal Chop | 20 x each side | 15 |
| 6 Diagonal Dorsal Loading | 20 x each side | 15 |
| 4 Exercise Band Abduction With Side Step | 20 x each side | 15 |
| 3 CLX Side Plank With Upper-Body Rotation | 15 x each side | 15 |
| 5 Medicine Ball Walkover | 20 x side to side | 15 |
| NOTE: Take a one- to two-minute break, and then repeat all the exercises. | | |

# 3.6 CROSSFIT WORKOUTS

## Exercise 1: 5-Degree Side Lunge ★ ★

Muscles trained: all muscle groups

Equipment: Gymstick Aerobic Bar

Procedure: Stand with the feet shoulder-width apart. Place the aerobic bar at the third lever arm. The upper arm is flexed from the shoulder joint and then again at the elbow joint. This provides proper static resistance. Perform the lunge as if you were moving around the face of a clock. First lunge to 1:00 position; second lunge to the 5:00 position; third lunge to the 7:00 position; and finally lunge to the 11:00 position. To get good neurological and proprioceptive results, do the lunges faster or change the lunge by starting with a different time.

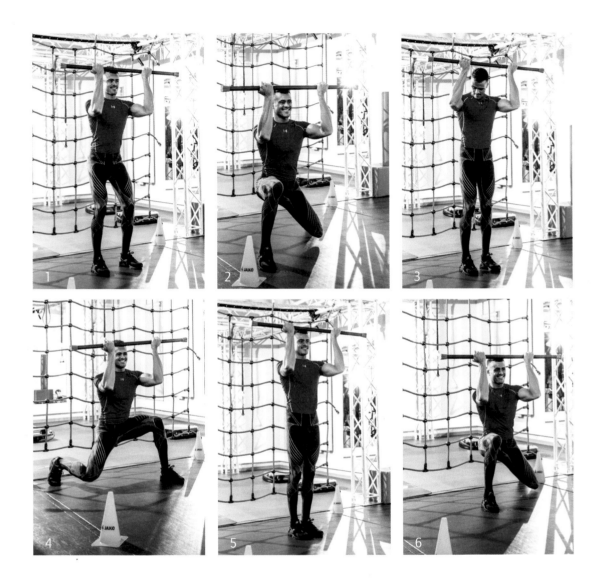

## Exercise 2:  CLX Flutter Kicks ★ ★ ★

Muscles trained: abs—legs

Equipment: TheraBand CLX, exercise mat

Procedure: Lie with your back on the mat in the supine position. Place the CLX bands on your feet. Place hands to the sides with the palms facing down. Raise one leg, keeping it as straight as your flexibility level allows. Try to get the leg perpendicular to the floor. Lower the leg and immediately raise with the other leg. Continue alternating legs. Keep looking up to avoid driving the chin toward the chest. Keep the shoulders retracted and back flat on the floor throughout the movement. Vary the pace and height of the kicks for a different intensity.

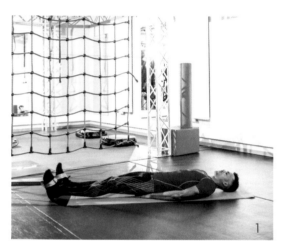
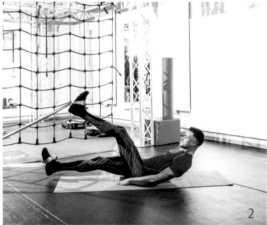

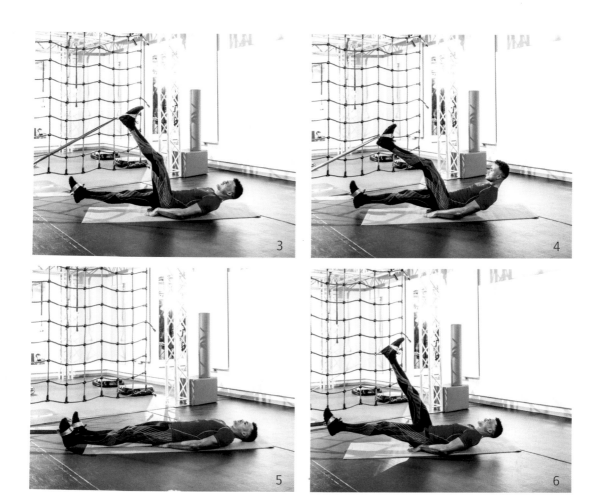

## Exercise 3: Medicine Ball 180-Degree Trunk Rotation With Lunge ★ ★ ★

Muscles trained: back—arms—shoulders—abs

Equipment: Medicine ball

Procedure: Stand with feet shoulder-width apart. Rotate the medicine ball to the right using the torso. Take a forward lunge while simultaneously bringing the medicine ball overhead as your torso turns 180 degrees. Bring the medicine ball all the way to the thigh or knee of the lunging leg.

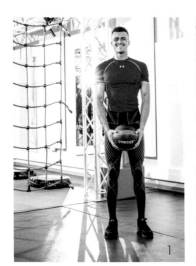
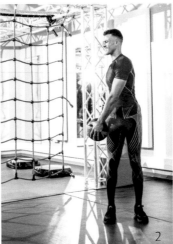
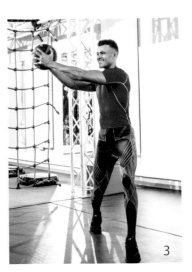

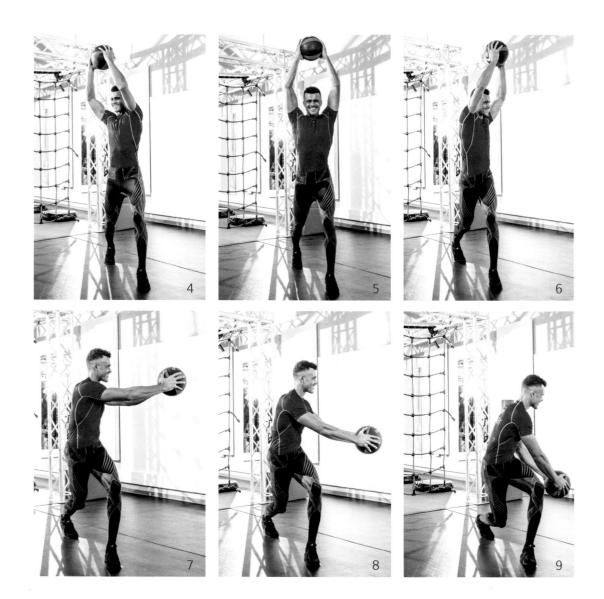

## Exercise 4:   Advanced Mini Ball Lying Twist ★ ★

Muscles trained: abs

Equipment: Mini exercise ball

Procedure: Lying on the floor with arms extended out to the side, lift your legs up with knees slightly bent. Grip the mini ball between your ankles. While keeping the mini ball in place, lower your legs to one side until the side of your thigh touches the floor. Raise your legs back to the starting position and repeat movement on the opposite side. Continue alternating sides for the desired repetitions.

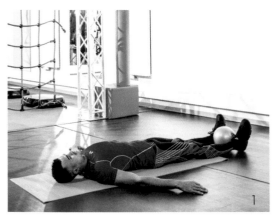
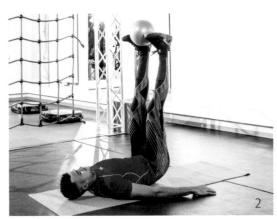
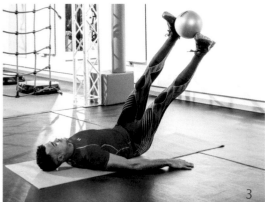
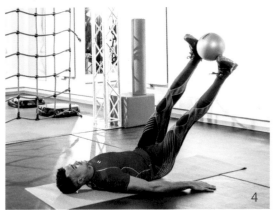

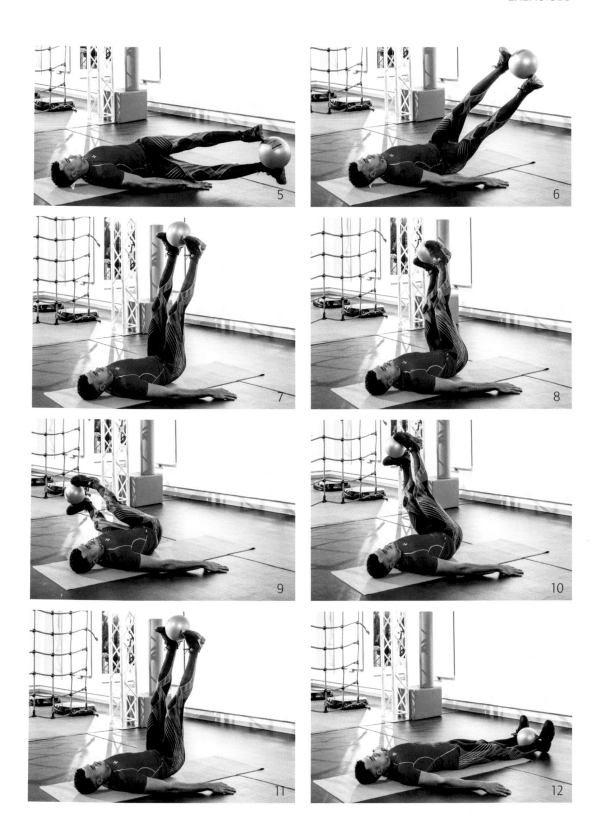

## Exercise 5:  Stability Ball Jackknife ★ ★ ★

Muscles trained: abs

Equipment: Stability ball, exercise mat

Procedure: Lie on the floor in a supine position and bring your arms up over your head. Grip the stability ball between your ankles. Raise your legs up, keeping the stability ball in place. At the same time, lift your upper body until it reaches your legs and stability ball. Pass the ball from your ankles to your hands. Return to the starting position and repeat, passing the ball from your hands to your ankles, and so on for desired repetitions.

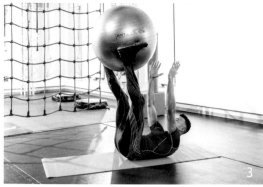

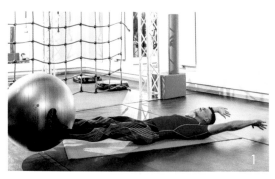

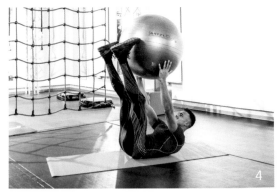

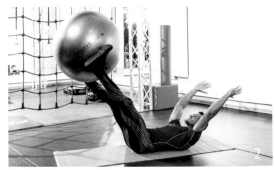

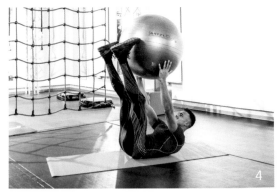

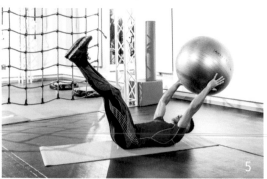

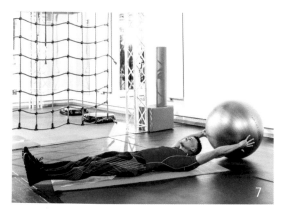

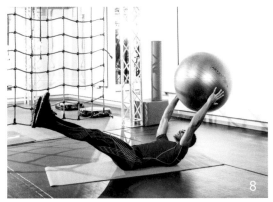

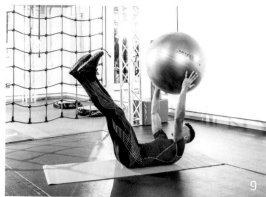

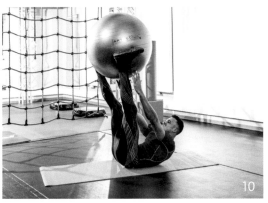

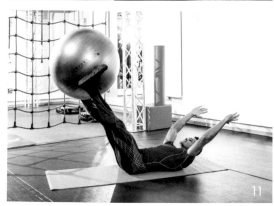

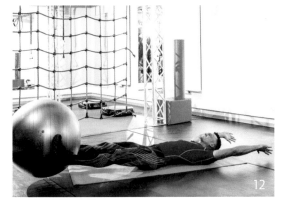

## Exercise 6:  Foam Roller Push-Up With Knee Flexion ★ ★

Muscles trained: abs–chest–shoulders–hips

Equipment: Foam roller

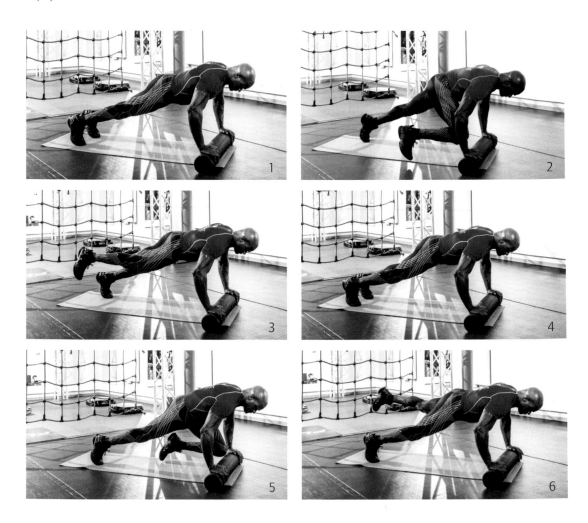

Procedure: Start in a push-up position with both hands on the foam roller. Both hands should be shoulder-width apart. Perform a push-up by flexing and extending the elbows. Bring one knee into the chest and then extend it behind you. Alternate bringing one knee into the chest and then extending the leg. It is important to hold the leg in the eccentric position for about 5 seconds. Return to the starting position and repeat.

## Exercise 7:  Foam Roller One-Arm Crossover  ★ ★ ★

Muscles trained: abs—obliques

Equipment: Foam roller

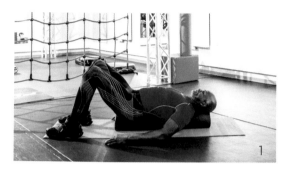
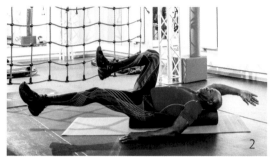
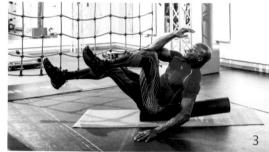
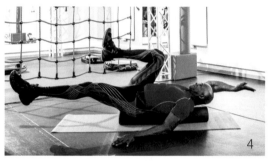
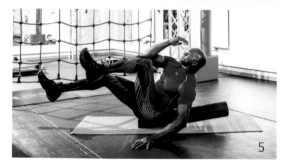
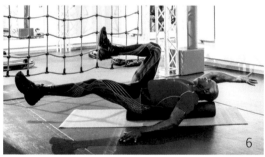

Procedure: Lie down with your vertebrae column on the foam roller. Make sure the neck and head are secure. Put your left arm down by your side and the right arm slightly beside your ear. With your back flat on the foam roller, extend the left leg and raise the heel from the floor. Your right leg is flexed at the knee with the foot off the floor. Then contralaterally curl and twist your torso, keeping the chin tilted up and the left hand on the floor. Slightly swing the right arm into the crossover by contralaterally moving the right elbow to the left knee. Return to the starting position and repeat for the desired repetitions before switching to the other side.

## Exercise 8: CLX Jumping Jack With Miniband ★ ★ ★

Muscles trained: all muscle groups

Equipment: TheraBand CLX, miniband

Procedure: Position the CLX band from behind and anchored high. Stand with legs and feet close together with the miniband positioned over the knees. Hold the CLX band down beside the hips. Lightly leap, spreading the legs approximately shoulder-width apart while simultaneously raising the arms overhead. Upon landing, immediately leap again, bringing the legs and arms back to the original starting position. Repeat in a continuous motion. Keep the core tight and head aligned with the spine. Vary the pace of the movement and the height of the jumps for different intensity levels.

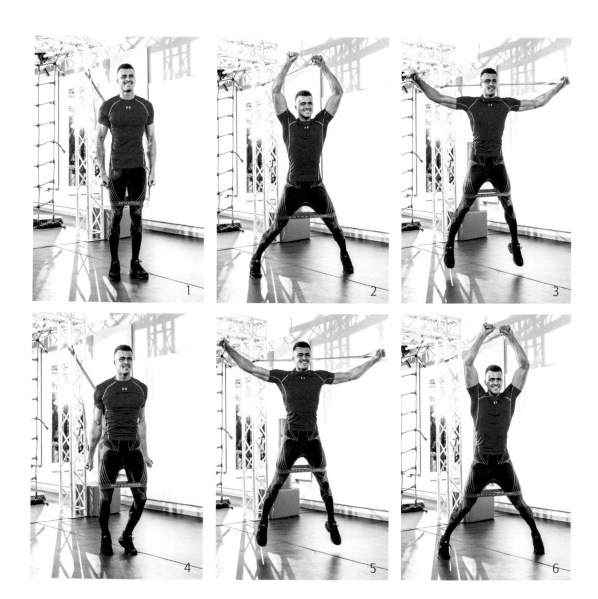

Using the previous eight exercises, perform circuit training two to three times a week for 20 to 30 minutes. There are two circuit variations, with circuit II being slightly more advanced than circuit I (see the following tables). The breaks between exercises should last only as long as needed to change position. This will ensure that the circuit training is effective.

## Circuit Training I

| EXERCISE | INTERVAL | REST (SECONDS) |
|---|---|---|
| 8 CLX Jumping Jack With Miniband | 15 sec | 15 |
| 2 CLX Flutter Kicks | 15 sec | 15 |
| 5 Stability Ball Jackknife | 15 sec | 15 |
| 4 Advanced Mini Ball Lying Twist | 15 sec | 15 |
| 6 Foam Roller Push-Up With Knee Flexion | 15 sec | 15 |
| 7 Foam Roller One-Arm Crossover | 15 sec | 15 |
| 3 Medicine Ball 180-Degree Trunk Rotation With Lunge | 15 sec | 15 |
| 1 45-Degree Side Lunge | 15 sec | 15 |
| NOTE: Take a one- to two-minute break, and then repeat all the exercises. | | |

CrossFit training can be short and effective when done using these eight exercises. It is a high-intensity, complex workout, giving you the maximum amount of benefits in the shortest amount of time. Generally, CrossFit workouts are designed as functional circuit training that can be done alone or in a small group.

## Circuit Training II

| EXERCISE | INTERVAL AND REPS | REST (SECONDS) |
|---|---|---|
| 8 CLX Jumping Jack With Miniband | 45 sec | 15 |
| 5 Stability Ball Jackknife | 45 sec | 15 |
| 2 CLX Flutter Kicks | 45 sec | 15 |
| 4 Advanced Mini Ball Lying Twist | 20 x side to side | 15 |
| 3 Medicine Ball 180-Degree Trunk Rotation With Lunge | 10 x per side | 15 |
| 1 45-Degree Side Lunge | 10 x per side | 15 |
| 6 Foam Roller Push-Up With Knee Flexion | 10 x per side | 15 |
| 7 Foam Roller One-Arm Crossover | 10 x per side | 15 |
| NOTE: Take a one- to two-minute break, and then repeat all the exercises. | | |

# 3.7 HIGH-INTENSITY INTERVAL TRAINING

### Exercise 1: Stability Ball Triceps Press ★ ★ ★

Muscles trained: shoulders—arms

Equipment: Stability ball

Procedure: Stand with your back to the stability ball. Place your hands on the ball behind your hips, slightly sideways and slanted. This position takes the pressure off of the wrists. Stabilize and contract your arms and back as well as your legs, moving away from the ball so that only your hands are contacting the ball. Then flex the elbows and lower your body down, supporting your weight with your arms, legs, and core. Return to the starting position and repeat.

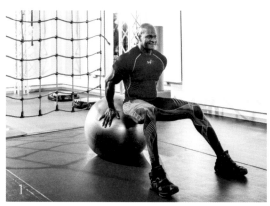
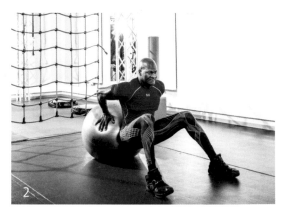
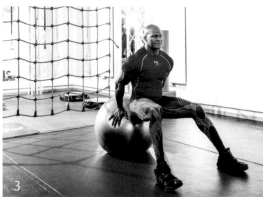

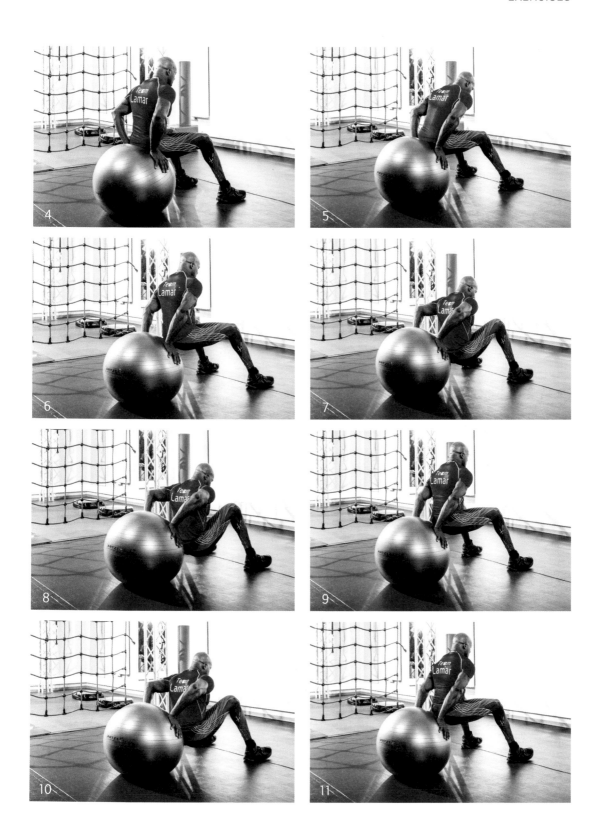

## Exercise 2:   CLX Mountain Climber  ★ ★ ★

Muscles trained: hips—back—shoulders—abs

Equipment: TheraBand CLX

Procedure: Put your feet through the loop of the CLX band that corresponds with your strength resistance level. Hold the CLX band between your thumb and the palm in the prone position. This position will stabilize the CLX band so it remains still. Start in the push-up position, hands shoulder-width apart and feet hip-width apart. Keep the head aligned with the spine and maintain a straight body position. Holding the push-up position, dynamically bring the knees to the chest, alternating legs as if you were running. Repeat for the desired number of repetitions.

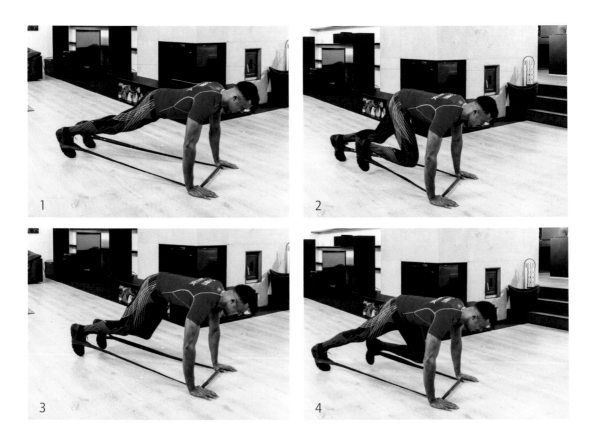

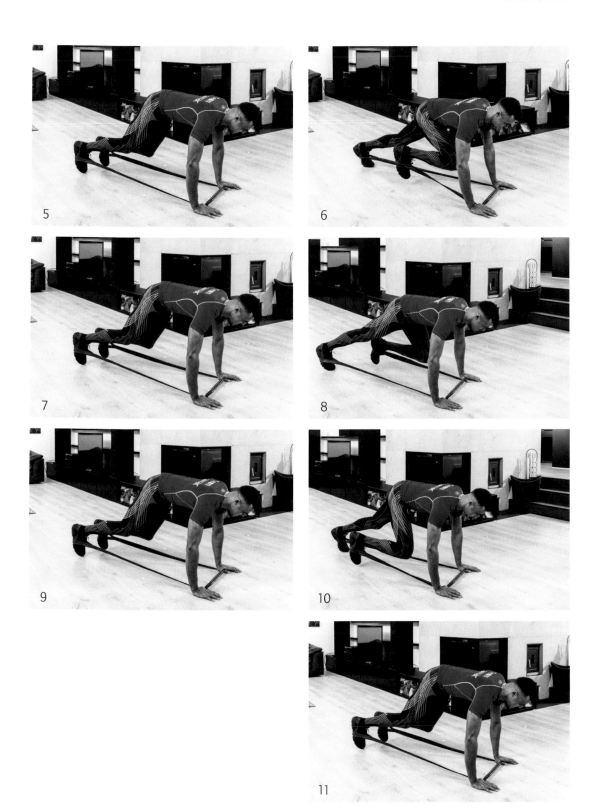

## Exercise 3:   Jumping Rope ★ ★ ★

Muscles trained: all muscle groups

Lower body: Though the calves are the main muscles powering the jump, your quadriceps, hamstrings, and glutes are also activated. The loading phase of rolling through the ball of your foot and pushing off with the toes uses the posterior side of your body, your glutes, hamstrings, and calves. The quadriceps and glutes help you control the jump and land lightly on your feet rather than hitting the floor with a thud. The knees should be slightly bent during both the push-off and landing phases of the jump.

Upper body: The shoulders and abs are the upper-body power muscles when jumping rope, though the arms and hands also help to swing the rope. Along with the core, your back stabilizes your upper body. The back should be elongated, straight, and centered over your pelvis rather than leaning forward or backward.

Equipment: Jump rope

Procedure: A high-intensity workout, jumping rope has long been a mainstay activity for boxers, professional athletes, and those wanting to increase their cardio endurance level. Along with building lean muscle mass by activating numerous muscle groups in both the lower and upper body, jumping rope is a calorie burner. Depending on your fitness level, jump rope for one to two minutes without stopping.

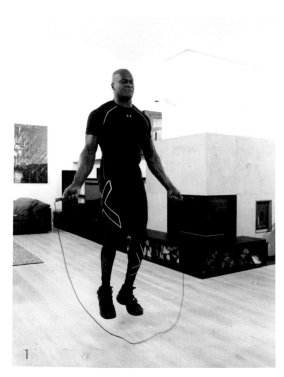

1

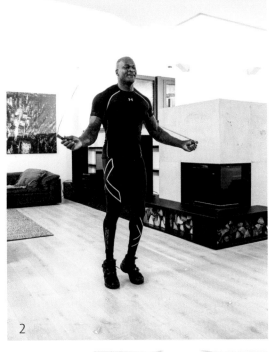

2

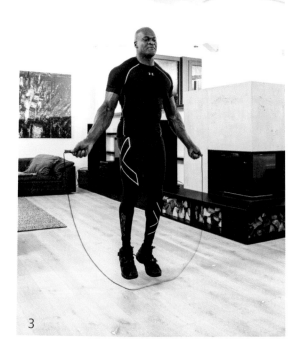

3

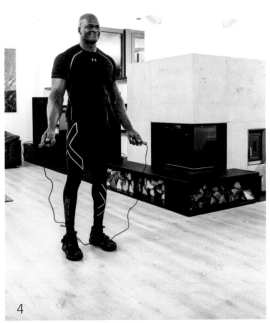

4

## Exercise 4:   Stability Ball Twister  ★ ★

Muscles trained: abs—shoulders—back—chest

Equipment: Stability ball

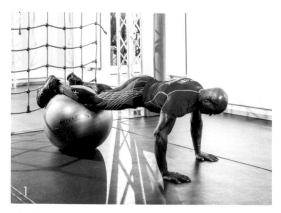

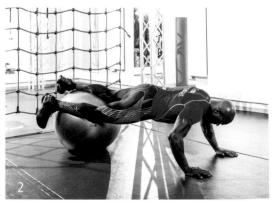

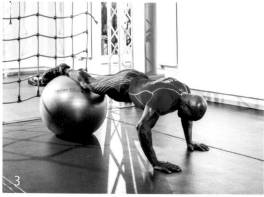

Procedure: Start in the push-up position with your feet on the stability ball and your hands on the floor. Position your legs and feet so that you can use them to grasp the stability ball. Keep your spine straight, and lightly contract the abdominal area. Begin to twist slightly at the pelvis; the pelvis, thighs, and legs act as a unit. Without moving the shoulders, go as far left and right as you can without losing the perfect form of the core from the shoulders to the knees. When you become adapted to the exercise, attempt to increase the speed.

## Exercise 5: CLX Jumping Jack ★ ★ ★

Muscles trained: abs—back—shoulders—legs

Equipment: TheraBand CLX

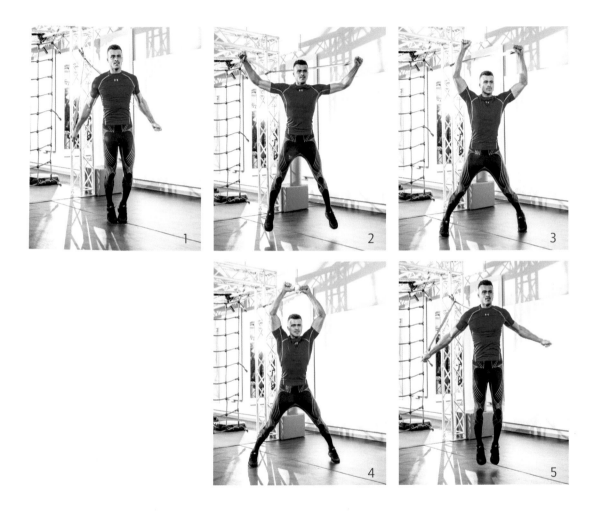

Procedure: Position the CLX band behind you and anchored high. Stand with the feet close together. Hold the CLX band in both hands down beside the hips. Lightly leap, so the legs are out to the side, approximately shoulder-width apart. Simultaneously raise the arms to the sides. Upon landing, immediately leap again, bringing the legs and arms back to the original starting position. Repeat in a continuous motion. Keep the core tight and head aligned with the spine. Vary the pace of the movement and the height of the jumps for different intensity levels.

## Exercise 6:   Kettlebell Lateral Arm Raise on Stability Ball ★ ★ ★

Muscles trained: shoulders—back

Equipment: Kettlebell, stability ball

Procedure: Lie with your side on a stability ball and position the feet one on top of the other on the ground to challenge balance. Using a neutral grip, hold the kettlebell down by the side of the stability ball. You should be using the hand opposite the side of the body that is on the stability ball. Use your other hand to provide further stability, placing it on the floor a little in front of the stability ball. Lift the kettlebell perpendicular to your body by fully extending your arm. Hold momentarily and return to the starting position. Repeat for desired repetitions and then switch and perform on the opposite side.

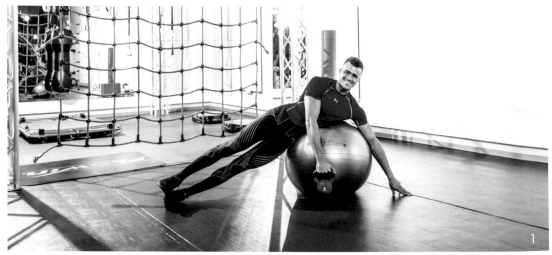

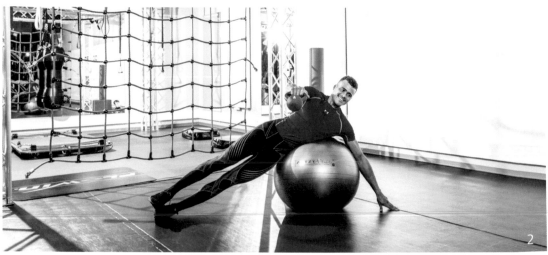

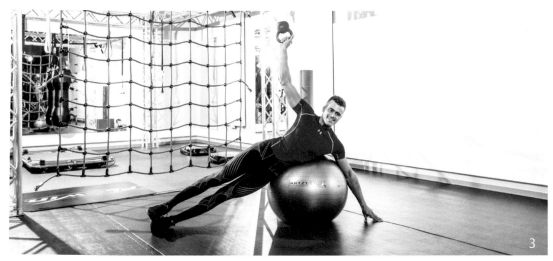

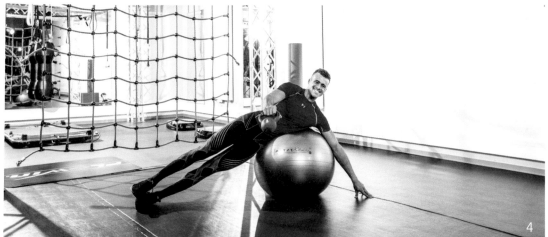

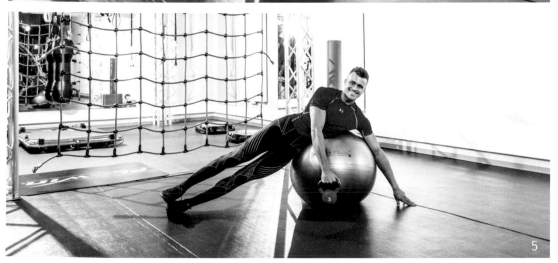

### Exercise 7: Kettlebell Side Step to Sumo Squat ★ ★ ★

Muscles trained: all muscle groups

Equipment: Kettlebell

Procedure: Stand with your feet shoulder-width apart. Reach down and pick up the kettlebell which should be positioned between your feet. Bring the kettlebell up to the chest as you hold it with both hands. Drop into the squat. Stay low and take a side step. Then go down onto the knees, one after the other. Get up, one leg at a time, and pause for a moment in the sumo squat position. Stand up and return to starting position and repeat. Be sure to perform equal repetitions in both directions.

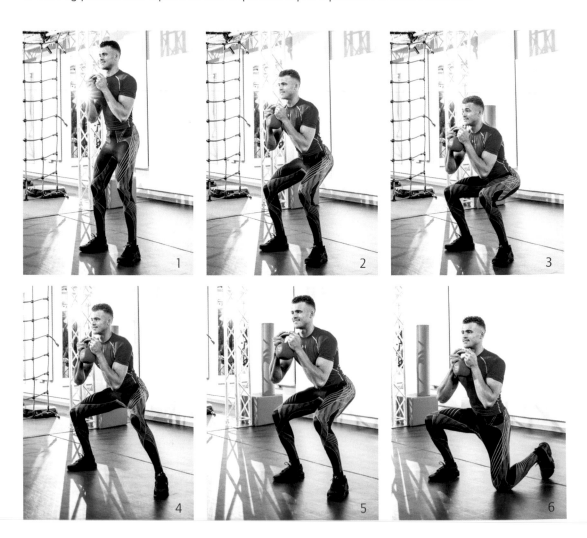

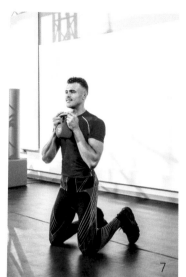

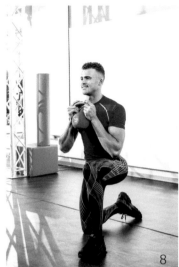

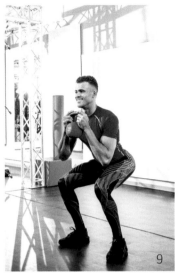

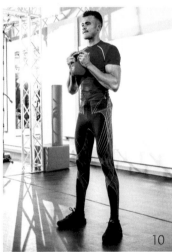

## Exercise 8: Stability Ball Pike ★ ★ ★

Muscles trained: all muscle groups

Equipment: Stability ball

Procedure: From a plank position with thighs on the stability ball, extend your legs straight behind you. Roll your shoulders back. Walk forward with your hands so the ball rests under your knees or the top of the feet, depending on how difficult you want the exercise to be. Push your hips up while pulling the stability ball closer to your chest. The ball should roll with you, helping to maintain stability. Return to the starting position and repeat.

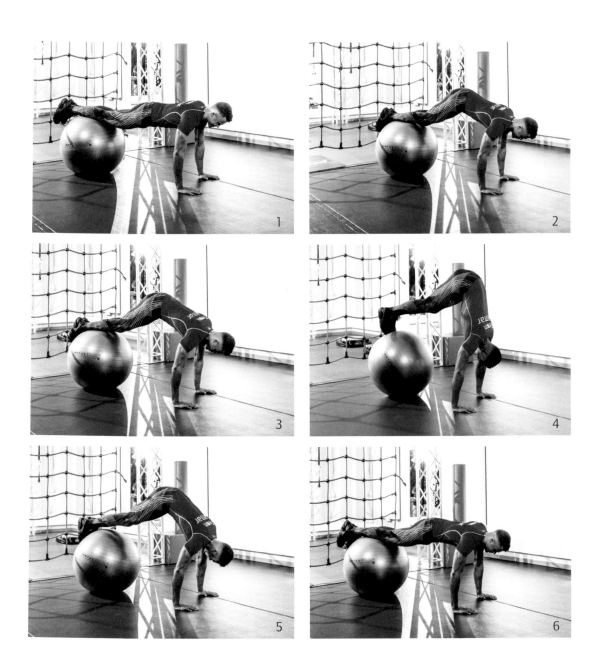

Using the previous eight exercises, perform circuit training two to three times a week for 20 to 30 minutes. There are two circuit variations, with circuit II being slightly more advanced than circuit I (see the following tables). The breaks between exercises should last only as long as needed to change position. This will ensure that the circuit training is effective.

## Circuit Training I

| EXERCISE | SETS AND REPS | REST (SECONDS) |
|---|---|---|
| 1 Stability Ball Triceps Press | 10x | 30 |
| 2 CLX Mountain Climber | 30 sec | 30 |
| 4 Stability Ball Twister | 30 sec | 30 |
| 5 CLX Jumping Jack | 30 sec | 30 |
| 7 Kettlebell Side Step to Sumo Squat | 30 sec | 30 |
| 3 Jumping Rope | 30 sec | 30 |
| 8 Stability Ball Pike | 30 sec | 30 |
| 6 Kettlebell Lateral Arm Raise on Stability Ball | 30 sec | 30 |
| NOTE: Take a one- to two-minute break, and then repeat all the exercises. | | |

## Circuit Training II

| EXERCISE | SETS AND REPS | REST (SECONDS) |
| --- | --- | --- |
| 2 CLX Mountain Climber | 45 sec | 15 |
| 5 CLX Jumping Jack | 45 sec | 15 |
| 1 Stability Ball Triceps Press | 20x | 15 |
| 4 Stability Ball Twister | 45 sec | 15 |
| 8 Stability Ball Pike | 45 sec | 15 |
| 7 Kettlebell Side Step to Sumo Squat | 45 sec | 15 |
| 6 Kettlebell Lateral Arm Raise on Stability Ball | 45 sec | 15 |
| 3 Jumping Rope | 45 sec | 15 |
| NOTE: Take a one- to two-minute break, and then repeat all the exercises. | | |

# 3.8   LEG, ARM, AND CORE WORKOUTS

The following exercises target these specific areas of the body—legs, arms, and core—for a more full-body workout.

### Exercise 1:   Medicine Ball Walkover  ★ ★

Muscles trained: chest–arms–shoulders–back

Equipment: Medicine ball

Procedure: Place the right hand on medicine which is positioned directly under your chest. Place your knees on a pillow or cushion. Keeping your core tight, inhale and lower your body as far as you can. Pause at the bottom and then push back up to the starting position while exhaling. Do not drop your hips! Head should stay in the same position from start to finish. Switch sides by placing the left hand on the ball together with the right hand, and then move the right hand to the floor under the shoulder. Keeping your core tight, inhale and lower your body as far as you can. Pause at the bottom and then push back up to the starting position while exhaling. Do not drop your hips! Repeat the exercise.

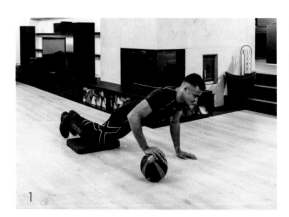
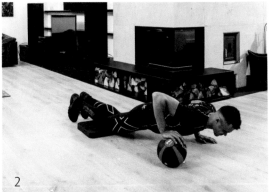

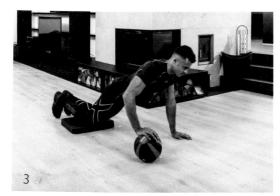

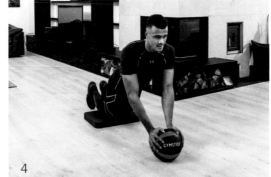

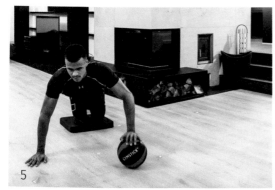

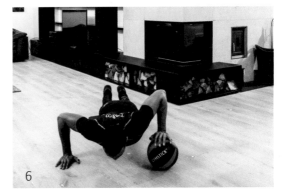

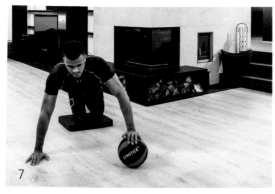

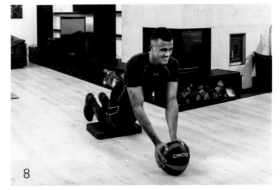

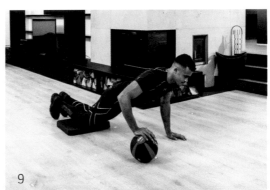

## Exercise 2:  Medicine Ball One-Arm Push-Up ★ ★ ★

Muscles trained: arms—back—abs—shoulders

Equipment: Medicine ball

Procedure: Place the right hand on medicine ball, which is positioned directly under your chest. Keeping your core tight, inhale and lower your body as far as you can. Pause at the bottom and then push back up to the starting position while exhaling. Do not drop your hips! Head should stay in the same position from start to finish. Then lift the left arm from extension into flexion into hyperextension as far as you can and hold for 2 or 3 seconds, keeping your core tight. Repeat on one side for desired repetitions before switching to the other side.

NOTE: This exercise is very advanced and should only be performed once you have mastered the regular push-up on the medicine ball.

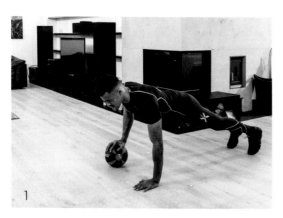
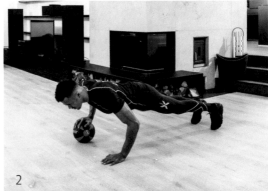

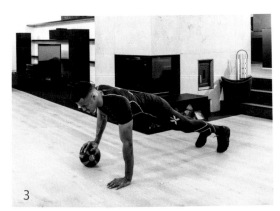

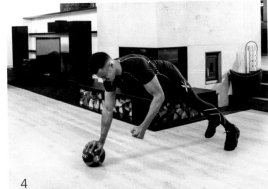

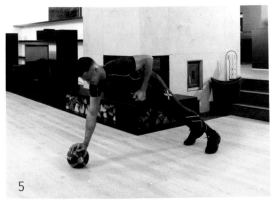

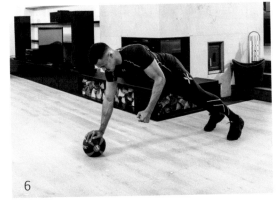

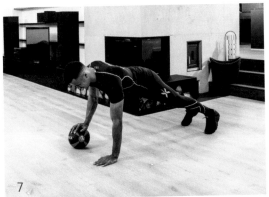

### Exercise 3: Foam Roller Jackknife ★ ★ ★

Muscles trained: abs

Equipment: Foam roller

Procedure: Lie with your vertebrae column on the foam roller. Make sure that neck and head are aligned and stable. Place the left arm down by your side and the right arm slightly beside your head. With your back flat on the foam roller and both legs extended with heels above the floor, perform a jackknife by curling your knees into the body, keeping the chin tilted up and the left hand on the floor. Slightly swing the right arm along the right side of the body all the way to the right knee. Extend your legs forward and your arm behind you and repeat. Once you have completed the desired repetitions, perform on the left side.

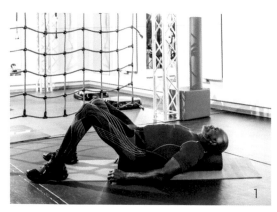
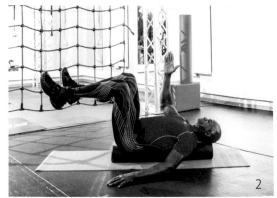
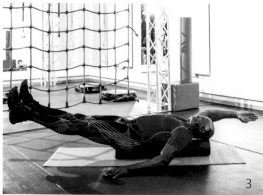
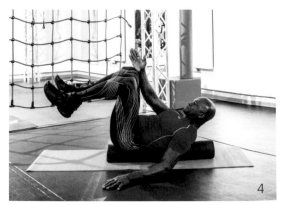

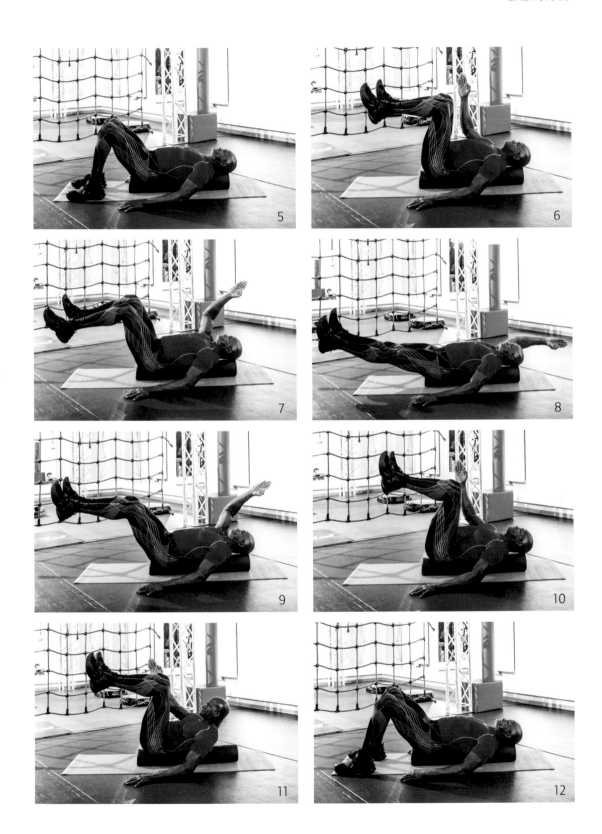

## Exercise 4:   Foam Roller One-Arm Crossover  ★ ★ ★

Muscles trained: abs

Equipment: Foam roller

Procedure: Lie down with your vertebrae column on the foam roller. Make sure that your neck and head are aligned and supported. Place the left arm down by your side and the right arm slightly beside your ear. With your back flat on the foam roller, extend your left leg and raise your heel away from the floor. Your right leg is flexed with the foot off the floor. Then contralaterally curl and twist your torso, keeping the chin tilted up and the left hand on the floor. With a slight swing, cross the right elbow contralaterally over to the left knee. Return to the starting position and then repeat. Once you have completed the desired repetitions, repeat on the left side.

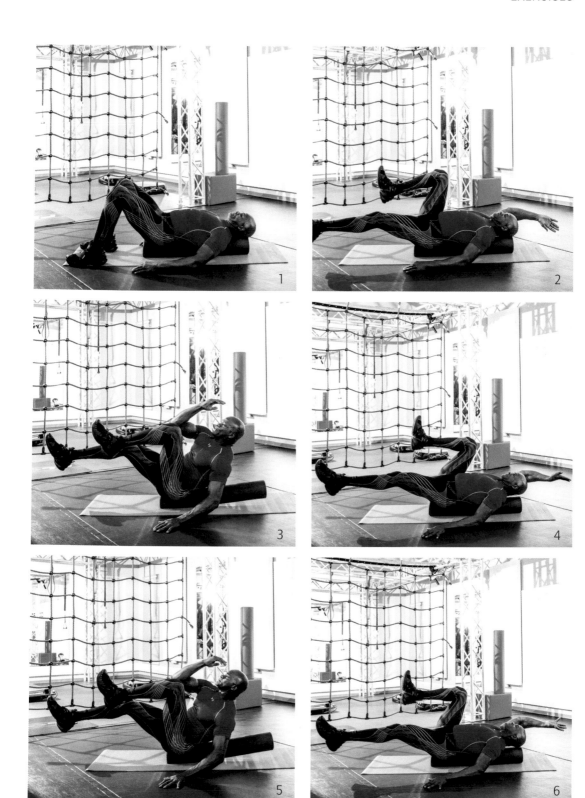

## Exercise 5:   Stability Ball Leg Curl  ★ ★ ★

Muscles trained: legs

Equipment: Stability ball, exercise mat

Procedure: Lie supine on floor with the lower legs on the stability ball. Extend arms out to sides. Raise your hips, bringing the lower back off floor. Lift the left leg about 60 degrees by flexing from the hip. Keeping the hips straight, bend the right knee, pulling the heel backward. Allow the foot to roll onto the ball. Lower to starting position by straightening the right knee and lowering the left leg. Repeat for desired repetitions and then repeat on the opposite side. Keep hips straight throughout the movement. Dorsal flexion of the ankle reduces insufficient movement of the gastrocnemius, allowing it to assist in knee flexion.

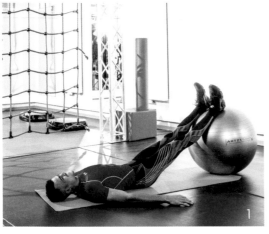
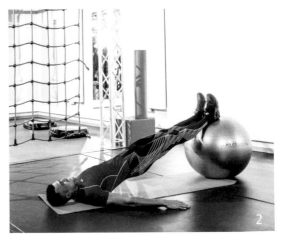
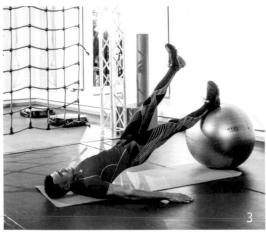
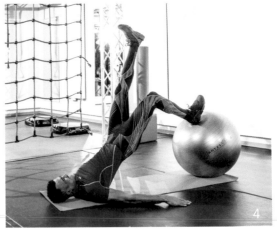

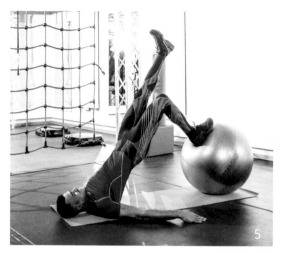

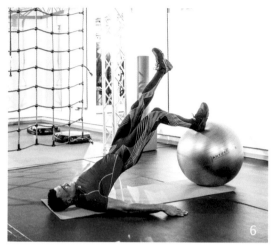

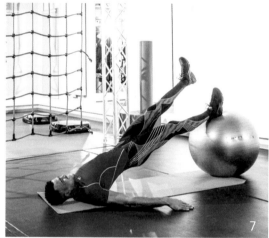

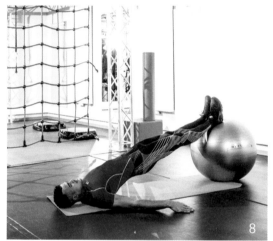

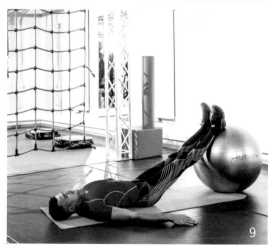

## Exercise 6:   Medicine Ball Squat Toss ★ ★

Muscles trained: legs

Equipment: Medicine ball

Procedure: Holding the medicine ball in front of you, lower into a squat. From the squat, jump up and toss the medicine ball overhead. Catch the medicine ball and return to starting position and repeat.

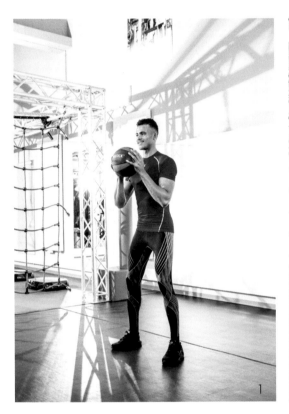
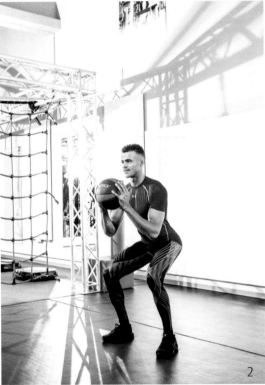

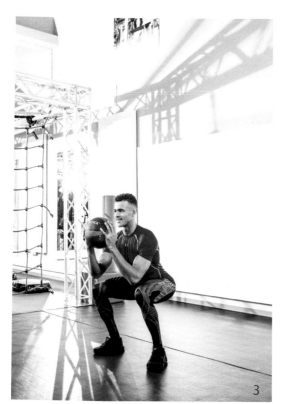

3

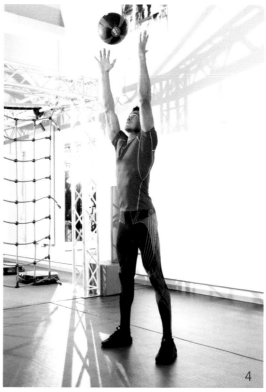

4

## Exercise 7: Stability Ball Triceps Press ★ ★ ★

Muscles trained: arms

Equipment: Stability ball

Procedure: Stand with your back to the stability ball. Place your hands slightly sideways and slanted on the stability ball. This takes the pressure off the wrists. Stabilize and contract your arms and back as well as your legs muscles and walk away from the ball. Only your hands should be touching the ball. Lower your body down by flexing at the elbows, supporting your weight with your arms, legs, and core. Return to the starting position and repeat.

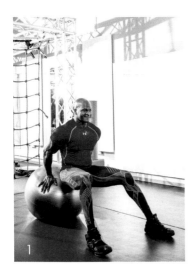
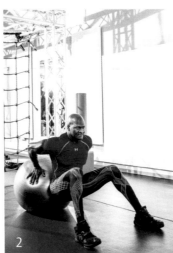
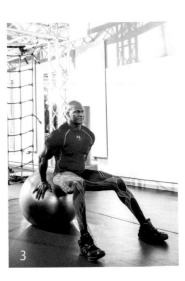

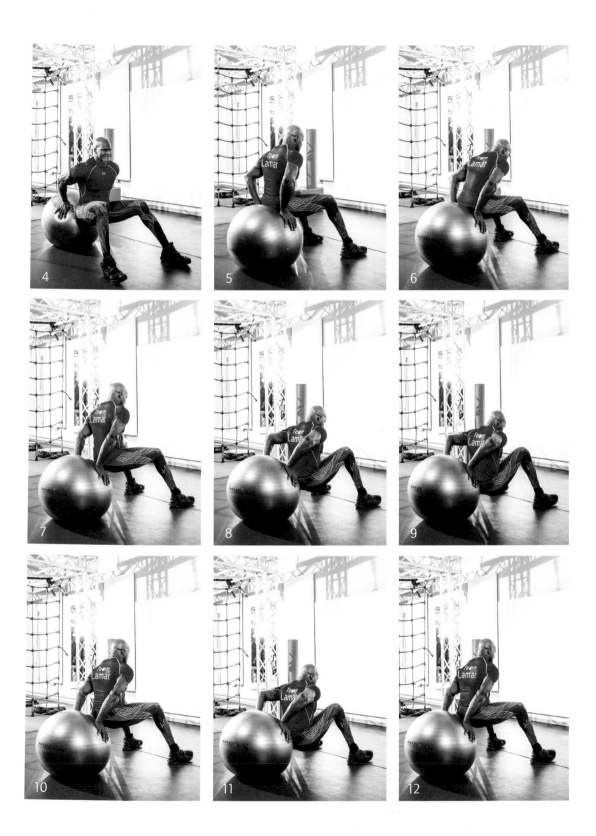

Using the previous seven exercises, perform circuit training two to three times a week for 20 to 30 minutes. There are two circuit variations, with circuit II being slightly more advanced than circuit I (see the following tables). The breaks between exercises should last only as long as needed to change position. This will ensure that the circuit training is effective.

## Circuit Training I

| EXERCISE | SETS AND REPS | REST (SECONDS) |
|---|---|---|
| 1 Medicine Ball Walkover | 10 x side to side | 30 |
| 2 Medicine Ball One-Arm Push-Up | 10 x each side | 30 |
| 3 Foam Roller Jackknife | 10 x each side | 30 |
| 4 Foam Roller One-Arm Crossover | 10 x each side | 30 |
| 5 Stability Ball Leg Curl | 10 reps | 30 |
| 6 Medicine Ball Squat Toss | 10 reps | 30 |
| 7 Stability Ball Triceps Press | 10 reps | 30 |
| NOTE: Take a one- to two-minute break, and then repeat all the exercises. | | |

## Circuit Training II

| EXERCISE | SETS AND REPS | REST (SECONDS) |
| --- | --- | --- |
| 6 Medicine Ball Squat Toss | 20x | 15 |
| 1 Medicine Ball Walkover | 20 x side to side | 15 |
| 2 Medicine Ball One-Arm Push-Up | 20 x each side | 15 |
| 4 Foam Roller One-Arm Crossover | 20 x each side | 15 |
| 3 Foam Roller Jackknife | 20 x each side | 15 |
| 7 Stability Ball Triceps Press | 20x | 15 |
| 5 Stability Ball Leg Curl | 20x | 15 |
| NOTE: Take a one- to two-minute break, and then repeat all the exercises. | | |

# 4 HOW TO MAKE BETTER FOOD CHOICES

"Eat your potatoes so you'll be full" is what my mother frequently said. She cooked from scratch every day. We often ate meat (my father loved meat and hearty food), and on Fridays we ate fish. We always had vegetables or a salad and potatoes. Pasta was something special, and we loved it as children. We ate most of our meals together—except for breakfast when my father buried himself in the newspaper and my mother was busy preparing school lunches for three children. While we ate, we talked about our day. There was always fresh fruit in our lunch boxes.

"Meat provides vital energy!" This old advertising slogan, coined and made popular by agricultural marketing companies during the 1970s, stood in direct contrast to the ongoing cholesterol debate. Scientists like Ancel Keys fed our guilty conscience with statements like: "A high-cholesterol diet with meat, eggs, and butter is the cause of coronary heart disease and heart attacks" (Seven Countries Study).

After my uncle's premature death from a heart attack in the 70s, we only used margarine instead of butter as a spreadable fat. And we increasingly heard things like: "Don't eat so much meat; it's unhealthy and has too much cholesterol."

By the time I studied ecotrophology in the 1980s, I had my own household and followed the lead of many of my fellow students. I ate a diet based on the rules of whole-food nutrition, meaning hardly any meat. And I learned: Science is fluid, and there are constantly new findings that must be taken into account.

During the 1990s, we began to hear those first voices that spoke of a "cholesterol lie," and one had to presume yesterday's findings are today's falsities.

The "proper diet." Is there such a thing? Which recommendations should one follow?

After decades of warnings from doctors regarding the excessive consumption of foods that contain cholesterol, the US did an about-face in 2015 and removed that passage from their dietary guidelines. The German Nutrition Society revised their fat guidelines in 2015 and wrote: "A reduction in fat intake is unnecessary as long as energy intake is controlled by observing long-term constant-weight considerations."

For decades, expert recommendations regarding nutrition were eat low fat and be calorie-conscious. And the consumption of low-fat and reduced-calorie (light) products really did go up, but people's weight also steadily increased. More than one in two adults (52%) in Germany are overweight. Men are affected more often than women: 62% of men are too heavy; 43% of women are overweight.

In the US, the percentage of overweight people has gone up from just over 40% in 1960 to more than 75%. (Since 1997, the percentage of obese people in the US has increased from 19% to roughly 34%.) Worldwide, every third person is overweight.

The affluent citizen eating a bad diet is often, but not exclusively, overweight or obese and also suffers from metabolic disorders: high blood pressure, diabetes, fat metabolism disorders, cardiovascular diseases, which are considered possible secondary diseases caused by excess weight.

Today, excess weight and obesity are still defined via BMI. Anyone with a BMI of between 25 and 29.9 is considered overweight. Values of 30 or higher indicate obesity or adiposity.

The body mass index (BMI) describes the relationship between body weight and height and is calculated based on the following formula:

Body weight (in kg) divided by height (in cm/m) squared

**Please note regarding BMI:** The body mass index offers only an initial rough estimate. For instance, people with lots of muscle mass can have a high BMI without being overweight. The BMI also does not offer information regarding the distribution of body fat. Excessive belly fat is considered a particular health risk. At this time, many experts, therefore, consider the **waist-to-height ratio (WHR)** to provide more meaningful data. Here a value of less than 0.5 (0.6 for older people) is considered desirable.

A median BMI of 22, an energy intake of 2,300 kcal for men and 1,800 for women between the ages of 25-50 (German Nutrition Society, 2015) is considered appropriate for healthy adults.

Athletes or people engaging in hard physical labor can certainly dispute this. Because the BMI tells us nothing about body composition—the percentage of muscle mass or fat distribution in the body. The latter is critical to the assessment of individual health risks.

## The basal metabolic rate (basic energy requirements) per day can be calculated using this simple formula:

For men: 1 kcal per 1 kg of body weight per hour

For women: 0.9 kcal per 1 kg body weight per hour

Energy requirements: Beginning at age 30, the basal metabolic rate decreases by approximately 3% per year. We must always take body composition into account. The general rule is: The larger the muscle mass, the higher the basal metabolic rate. The explanation is simple. Muscle tissue has a considerably higher metabolic rate than fat.

So what is the right diet? Which recommendations should one follow to stay thin, fit, and productive? Never have there been more choices than today, but that is also true for the amount of confusion. Lots of meat or only a little; vegetarian or even vegan? A lot or a little bread, pasta, and potatoes? Which fats are the right ones, and how much fat should one consume?

**Vegetarians:** The vegetarian diet foregoes animal products such as meat, meat products, and most often also fish. The consumption of milk, milk products, and eggs makes ovo-lacto vegetarianism a balanced version of a vegetarian diet.

**Pescetarians** also eat fish.

**Vegans** forego all animal products, even honey, and do not wear clothing made from animal products, such as wool, leather, and silk.

Being interested in healthy food or eating a balanced diet can sometimes be complicated. Contradictions, changing recommendations, and the vast offerings in stores confuse the consumer as much as the constant new foods, beverages, and nutritional supplements do. Add to that reports about rotten meat and food scandals.

Today's foods are often very high in calories. Before we are even satiated, we have already consumed more calories than we need. The potato, as I ate it in my childhood, is still popular with consumers. Not as the classic boiled potato, but rather as chips, French fries, or croquettes. Humans lack instincts when it comes to their diet.

A balanced diet represents health, fitness, and productivity. But what exactly is a balanced diet?

Our nutritional experts offer us official recommendations. The German Nutrition Society compiles reference values for dietary guidelines. According to German experts, people should consume lots of carbohydrates, meaning at least 50% of the total energy intake (GNS 50-60%), moderate amounts of protein (0.8g/kg of body weight) or 10% of the energy intake, and little fat, 30% maximum of consumed calories.* In the food industry, the offerings of light, low-fat, or reduced-calorie products are vast. But the bodyweight trend in the population is alarming. Is it possible that our current dietary guidelines are based on outdated findings, and that new findings are being ignored?

Since the 1970s in the US, the amount of calories from fat consumed daily has dropped from 45% to 34%. At the same time, the average amount of carbohydrates rose from 39% to 51%. This created a 250kcal increase per day. Simultaneously, people were becoming less physically active.

## Nutritional Building Blocks

Our nutrition is made up of different building blocks. For our main meals, we typically choose one component from each building block. We put emphasis on the water-rich foods like vegetables and fruit, combined with proteins such as fish, meat, dairy, and eggs. We supplement with whole grains—sparingly and based on personal lifestyle—like bread, pasta, or potatoes. Fats like butter, high-grade oils, or nuts complete our meals.

*German Nutrition Society: Reference values for dietary guidelines

# 4.1   CARBOHYDRATES

## What Are Carbohydrates?

- Carbohydrates are one of the main nutrients along with protein and fat.

- They provide 4 kcal per gram.

- They provide quick energy.

- They come primarily from grain products, potatoes, and sweets.

Carbohydrates provide quick energy from starches in bread, potatoes or pasta, and sweets. Starch is, in simplified terms, a concatenation of many glucose building blocks.

The muscles and the brain are generally the primary consumers of carbohydrates in the form of glucose.

## Do We Have to Eat Carbohydrates?

Since our bodies are able to build glucose during metabolism, we are not essentially dependent on carbohydrates from food.

## What Happens in the Body After a Carbohydrate-Rich Meal?

As starch moves through our digestive system, it is divided into its individual building blocks, glucose. The glucose is reabsorbed into the blood (we can measure this as an increase in blood sugar) from where it is channeled to the muscle cells and brain cells and is available for energy production.

We require insulin as the "door opener" to the somatic cells. This hormone from the pancreas becomes active whenever we eat carbohydrates and our blood sugar level rises after a meal. But our muscle cells can only absorb limited amounts of glucose. This varies depending on lifestyle. The more energy is burned in the muscle cell, the more supply—glucose—is absorbed. This means that people who move a lot, are active in everyday life, exercise, or do physically strenuous work require a greater energy supply in the form of carbohydrates, and they burn more carbohydrates. Someone who drives to work, uses the elevator, spends the day sitting at his desk, and ends the day on the sofa watching television burns little energy in the muscles. Once the muscles' glucose absorption capacity is exhausted, the excess of consumed carbohydrates accumulates outside the muscle cell in the form of glucose. Here there is only one way out: the fat cell. With the help of insulin, the excess sugar is then channeled to the fat cells, converted to fat, and stored for hard times—in the form of love handles.

Those who eat a lot of carbohydrates program their metabolism to store fat. Insulin promotes fat buildup while also hindering fat reduction. Insulin is a fat storage hormone, or simply a "fat hormone."

People who don't get much exercise as well as overweight people, particularly those with a large girth, should consume carbohydrates sparingly (low-carb diet). In these people, insulin is usually less effective (insulin resistance), which results in a higher insulin release from the pancreas to compensate for the lack of effectiveness. In overweight people, these higher insulin releases result in additional fat storage (weight gain) and make it more difficult to lose weight. The fat hormone makes a good job of it. Stress, sleep deprivation, and menopause in women are all factors that speak for a low-carb diet. Bread, pasta, and potatoes are not a problem for thin, active people without belly fat.

In general, the preferred choice should be "slow" carbs that are released more slowly into the blood: whole-grain products and, of course, water-rich carbohydrates in the form of vegetables.

Here is an easy way to reduce carbohydrates:

*Table 4: Carbohydrate alternatives*

| INSTEAD OF... | ...IT'S BETTER TO HAVE |
| --- | --- |
| Juice mixed with water | Water with fruit slices |
| 1 slice white bread (2 oz.) | 1 thin slice of whole-grain bread (1 oz.) |
| 4 oz. noodles, cooked | 2 oz. noodles + 2 oz. vegetable spaghetti |
| 1 oz. muesli | 1 oz. chopped nuts |
| 5 oz. fruit yogurt | 5 oz. plain yogurt + fresh fruit |
| Jam | Fruit spread |
| Milk chocolate | Semi-sweet chocolate |

TIP: Carbohydrates rich in starch and sugar should be consumed only sparingly in order to get as little fat storage hormone as possible. The right carbohydrate, such as whole grains, natural rice, or whole-grain noodles, are only consumed in moderation. They flow more slowly into the blood and release a lower insulin response. Quickly available carbohydrates from soft drinks and sweets should generally be avoided. In general, the less sugar (including fruit sugar), the better.

## Sample One-Day, Low-Carb Menu for Weight Loss

### Breakfast

- Slice of whole-grain bread (19 g carbs)
- 2 oz. ham (0 g)
- Coffee + 3 oz. milk (5 g)
- 1 bell pepper (11 g)
- 1 Tbs. butter (–)

Total: 35 g of carbohydrates

### Lunch

- 7 oz. steak (0 g)
- 11 oz. spinach (2 g)
- 2 Tbs. olive oil (0 g)

### Snack

- Slice of cheese (0 g)
- 1 apple (14 g)

Total: 16 g of carbohydrates

### Dinner

- 2-egg omelet (1 g)
- 9 oz. tomato–cucumber salad (4 g)
- 1 Tbs. butter (0 g)
- 1 Tbs. rapeseed oil (0)
- 1 kiwi

Total: 10 g of carbohydrates

Total carbohydrates for the day: 61 g

# 4.2 PROTEIN

## What Is Protein?

Proteins are necessary for the body's endogenous protein production. They include

- enzymes,

- hormones,

- muscles, and

- connective tissue.

Dietary protein provides 4 kcal per gram and is essential to humans. The body must ingest it with food because it is unable to produce certain amino acids (tiny protein building blocks).

## Where Do We Get Our Protein?

Protein sources include fish, lean meat, eggs, dairy (milk, cheese, plain yogurt, cottage cheese), and legumes as plant-based protein. Protein sources should vary daily and should be consumed with each meal, even snacks. A good choice here would be cottage cheese or plain yogurt combined with a little fruit salad or with raw veggie sticks.

## Proteins Are Our Substantial Foods

Proteins make us feel full and curb the rise of blood sugar levels. When the protein intake goes up the same time the carbohydrate intake goes down, the blood sugar level doesn't go up as much after a meal. This is a way to keep insulin levels relatively low (little fat hormone), which results in a lower fat storage rate. At the same time, we are less hungry, or rather feel less famished, because our blood sugar fluctuates less.

People who eat a varied vegetarian diet supply their bodies with the essential proteins through dairy, eggs, and legumes (plant protein). A vegan diet is only practical with lots of detailed knowledge and much effort. Good sources of protein for vegans are primarily legumes (also as sprouts). As a vegan, covering one's protein demands is difficult. A vegan diet is not recommended for children and pregnant women. Supplements like vitamin B12, vitamin D, calcium, and iodine are generally indispensable for vegans.*

*Nutrition survey from April 2016.

Problematic is the distribution of large quantities of ready-made vegan foods and meat substitute products. Inferior raw materials and lots of additives make these products questionable alternatives.

TIP: Integrate protein into every meal—for example, cottage cheese with breakfast, plain yogurt as a snack, meat (high-quality meat from species-appropriate husbandry, preferably grass-fed), fish (preferably farmed organic), eggs, or legumes with main meals. Heavily processed foods like cold cuts or fast food should be avoided because, in addition to the many additives, they often also contain sugar and fructose as undesirable ingredients.

# 4.3　FAT

## What Is Fat?

Dietary fats are important energy suppliers. The energy value of fat is more than twice as high as that of carbohydrates and proteins. At 9 kcal/g, fat has the highest energy density among the major nutrients (protein and carbohydrates have only 4 kcal/g). Fat is also a building block for various somatic cells, is indispensable as a solvent for fat-soluble vitamins, and uncontested as a provider of flavor and aroma for any food.

Fat must be consumed with food. We must consume certain essential fatty acids because they are vital but our bodies are unable to produce them. We particularly need a more beneficial ratio of pro-inflammatory omega-6 to anti-inflammatory omega-3 fatty acids in our diet. For this reason, we should consume plant-based oils made from flaxseed, walnuts, and rapeseed every day, while avoiding oils made from sunflowers, corn, and thistles. Meat from factory farms should be replaced with high-quality meat from species-appropriate husbandry because it contains a better fatty acid pattern.

Meanwhile, many studies have not confirmed the notion that saturated fats from meat, milk, and butter increase the risk of heart attack and stroke.

The perception that "fat makes fat" is still deeply rooted in the minds of consumers, and across the board, animal fats are considered unhealthy. The result: Decades of avoiding fat has made us fat, because avoiding fat has led to weight-gain from starches and sugar.

## Disarming Fats

People who like to eat fat should not worry about gaining weight. The high-energy density of fat can be mitigated with water-rich foods. The more water-rich a meal, the less weight fat carries. So for example, you should not put a high-fat cheese on dry bread, but rather enjoy it with a big salad or a vegetable stir-fry (lots of water).

A lot of fat along with carbohydrates (croissants, pasta with cream sauce, deep-fried, breaded) are not only energy-dense combinations, but are also bad for the figure. They should be avoided.

## Are Some Fats Unhealthy?

Yes, factory-made plant-based fats that have been hardened are unhealthy. Fat-hardening was used for decades in the production of margarine to turn liquid vegetable oil into a spreadable fat. This process creates transfats that are extremely questionable when it comes to health, particularly with respect to heart health. Today, the margarine industry uses a number of other production methods, but hardened fats are still frequently used in processed foods. Hardened fats should be avoided.

*Energy density* is the amount of energy a food or meal contains (in kcal or kj) per 3.5 oz. Foods with an energy density of less than 100 kcal/3.5 oz. are considered low-energy density foods. Medium-energy density would be up to 225 kcal per 3.5 oz., and > 225 per 3.5 oz. is considered high-energy density.

TIP: Instead of eating light, change your oils. Avoid sunflower, thistle, and corn oil (as well as margarine made from these oils), and instead alternate between

- flaxseed, rapeseed, and walnut oil (plant omega-3 FA);
- nuts, preferably walnuts;
- fatty fish like salmon, herring, mackerel (animal omega-3 FA);
- grass-fed meat (favorable omega-3 to omega-6 ratio);
- dairy products with a natural fat content, but unsweetened;
- olive oil; and
- butter as a spreadable fat.

Each meal should include a high-quality fat component. Avoid carbohydrate–fat bombs and hardened fats as well as foods that contain them.

# 4.4 DRINKS

In terms of quantity, water is the most important component of the human body and makes up 50-60% of body weight. The body's total amount of water varies depending on age, body fat percentage, and body weight.

Water has important functions within the body:

- Water maintains body temperature.

- All metabolic processes in our bodies take place in a watery environment.

- It transports nutrients and works as a solvent, including oxygen supply.

- Water is important for physical performance and concentration ability.

- It boosts our digestion.

- Water affects blood pressure.

## How Much Water Should I Drink?

Under normal conditions, we lose 78 oz. of water a day through urine, respiration, skin, perspiration, and stools. In warm weather, that water loss increases to 111 oz. During hard physical labor, that loss can be as high as 223 oz.

Under normal conditions, the body produces 10 oz. of water during oxidation processes; 34 oz. should be consumed via water-rich foods (vegetables, fruit). That is a total of 44 oz. If we now drink 34 oz. via beverages like water and tea, we have found a balance (78 oz.). Add a cushion amount of 17 oz., and the recommendation is to drink 51 oz. of fluid per day (under normal conditions).

## Symptoms of dehydration

1%   →   sensation of thirst

4%   →   diminished strength performance

5%   →   higher heart rate, cramps

10%   →   mental disturbances

15%   →   death

When we don't drink enough, our body does not get enough oxygen and nutrients. The lack of oxygen causes exhaustion. Toxins are not flushed out, and with prolonged dehydration, our blood pressure rises.

Water is the most important beverage. Today, tea and even coffee can be included as beverages as long as they are unsweetened. Lemonade, soft drinks, milk, and alcoholic beverages are no longer considered beverages. They are considered liquid food.

Sweetened beverages of any kind are not recommended. The large amounts of sugar elicit lots of the fat storage hormone insulin. But these sweet drinks do not satiate because they rush through our digestive tract and don't linger in the stomach. On the contrary, sweetened beverages make you hungry because the blood sugar level acts like a rollercoaster, and the quick drop in the blood sugar curve due to insulin causes you to feel ravenous.

Soft drinks, as well as unsweetened fruit juices, contain lots of fructose. Although it is metabolized without insulin, when it reaches the liver, it has to be further processed there since the liver cannot store fructose. When you consume a lot of fructose, it is transformed into fat and stored. This results in fatty liver as well as increased belly fat.

While diabetics were practically fattened up with fructose during the 1990s because it was thought that fructose was the perfect sugar for diabetics, today we know that fructose had dramatic consequences. Next to nonalcoholic fatty liver, another result is impaired fat metabolism function in the form of higher triglycerides. This promotes an increase in uric acid and gout.

## Are Drinks Sweetened With Artifical Sweeteners an Alternative?

Scientists continue to disagree when it comes to artificial sweeteners. Theories and disproven theories regularly take turns here. Reports like, for instance, "artificial sweeteners cause cancer" or "artificial sweeteners make you gain weight" are just a few of them.

For certain is that artificial sweeteners are very to extremely sweet. People who regularly consume beverages or foods sweetened with artificial sweeteners keep their sweetness threshold high, meaning the amount of sweetness they require to find something pleasantly sweet is kept at a high level. The goal should be to keep the sweetness threshold low and to sensitize one's taste buds to sweetness. Artificial sweeteners are generally synthetic products and must be detoxified by the body. It is everyone's personal choice: How much chemistry do I want to put in my body?

TIP: Nothing works without water! It is recommended to drink a glass of water every one to two hours. Avoid any kind of sweetened beverages and forego soft drinks and beverages containing fructose. Fruit juices and smoothies should be on the menu only occasionally! Fruit teas and herbal teas are a nice alternative.

# 4.5 VEGETABLES AND FRUIT

Vegetables are always good. An abundance of nutrients such as vitamins, minerals, and secondary plant substances provide a marvelous health cocktail. The high water content of these foods makes them ideal substantial foods. Our stomach is full, which activates the food satiation hormones, but at the same time we consume hardly any calories. The plentiful dietary fiber keeps the blood sugar level stable and has a positive effect on bowel function.

## Eat a Rainbow

"Eating lots of water" is our motto. With three vegetable servings per day, we can keep the energy density of a meal low. Selection is based on seasonal offerings and should be as colorful as possible. One serving is approximately one handful; for leaf lettuce, it is two handfuls. Vegetables can be eaten in generous amounts, and portion sizes can be increased if necessary.

According to research, three servings of vegetables and two servings of fruit per day can lower the risk of heart attack and stroke and protect us from colon cancer.

We limit fruit to two servings (handfuls). Experts even caution against excessive fruit consumption because of the negative effects of fructose on the body. Fruit should be eaten rather than drunk. Regularly drinking fruit juices and fruit smoothies can quickly become too much of a good thing because, for instance, that fresh-squeezed orange juice at breakfast has easily five oranges in it. Would we normally eat five oranges for breakfast?

Smoothies, preferably as a green version with less fruit and an additional vegetable serving, are a nice alternative.

TIP: Eat three large servings of vegetables, salad, and mushrooms and two servings of low-sugar fruit each day, which equals five a day. Make sure these water-rich foods are as colorful and versatile as possible. Vegetables and fruit lower the energy density of your meals and really fill you up. Make your selections based on seasonal offerings. Fresh or frozen products (without additives) are preferable.

# 4.6  RECIPES

## Fillet of Smoked Trout on Pumpernickel Bread

**Makes 4 servings**

- 9 oz. smoked trout fillets
- 2 dill sprigs
- 1/4 bunch of chives
- 2 Tbs. horseradish cream
- 5 oz. cream cheese

- 1-2 Tbs. whole-grain mustard
- A little salt, freshly ground black pepper
- 1-2 Tbs. lemon juice
- Pumpernickel bread (cucumber slices as a low-carb alternative)

### Preparation

1. In a bowl, combine horseradish, cream cheese, and mustard and stir until smooth.
2. Wash herbs, shake off excess water, and finely chop. Add to cream-cheese mixture.
3. Separate fish into small pieces (remove bones), add to cream-cheese mixture, and carefully fold in.
4. Add pepper and lemon juice to taste. If necessary, add a little salt.
5. Spread the cream-cheese mixture onto the pumpernickel bread. Cucumber slices are a good alternative as a low-carb version for fewer carbohydrates.

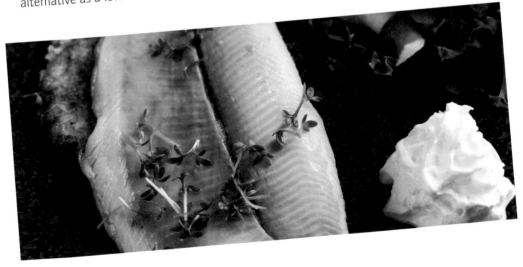

## Green Smoothie

Makes 2 servings

- 1 1/2 oz. of spinach leaves (fresh or frozen)—you can also use mache, arugula, regular lettuce
- 5 mint leaves
- 5 basil leaves
- 2 sprigs of parsley

- 1 small banana, peeled
- 1 apple, unpeeled and quartered
- 3 1/2 oz. orange juice
- 7 oz. water
- 1 Tbs. rapeseed oil

Preparation

1. Combine all ingredients and mix in a blender or with an immersion blender until finely pureed. The consistency varies based on the performance of your appliance.

Ingredients can be changed according to personal taste—for example, less fruit, more herbs and lettuce. Add some nuts or almonds. Use flavorful nut oils like walnut oil.

TIP: For an iced smoothie, use frozen spinach or ice water or ice cubes (if you have a sufficiently high-powered blender).

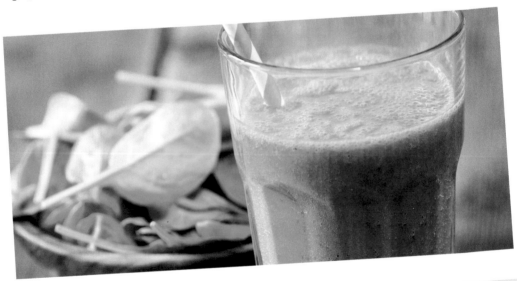

## Couscous Vegetable Salad

Makes 4 servings as an appetizer or 2 servings as a main course

- 1/3 cup instant couscous
- 3 oz. vegetable broth, pepper, cayenne pepper
- 1 head of romaine lettuce or another type of leaf lettuce
- 3 oz. of cherry tomatoes
- 1/4 salad cucumber
- 1/2 avocado

- 1 green onion
- 2 sprigs Italian parsley
- 6 oz. feta cheese
- 1 oz. tomato juice
- 1 Tbs. lemon juice
- 2 Tbs. olive oil
- Salt and pepper to taste

### Preparation

1. Pour the hot vegetable broth over the couscous and let it stand for 10 minutes.
2. Cut lettuce, cucumber, and avocado into small pieces; cut cherry tomatoes in half; finely cut spring onion; and combine all of these ingredients in a bowl and carefully fold under the cooled couscous.
3. Finely chop the parsley and add to mixture.
4. For the dressing, combine tomato juice, lemon, and oil and add to the salad.
5. Add pepper, cayenne pepper, and salt to taste.

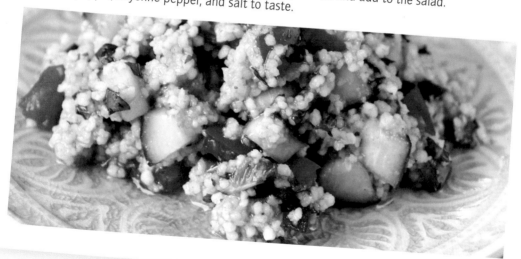

## Thai Chicken With Coconut Milk

**Makes 4 servings**

- 1 1/4 lb. chicken breast fillets cut into strips
- 2 Tbs. of rapeseed oil or nut oil (e.g., sesame)
- 1/4 Tsp. turmeric
- 1/4 Tsp. cumin
- 2 pinches coriander

- 1/4-1/2 Tsp. salt
- Pepper to taste
- 2 scallions
- 5 oz. carrots, sliced
- 7 oz. zucchini, sliced
- 7 oz. fennel, cut into pieces
- 1-2 garlic cloves

**Sauce**

- 1 14-oz. can of coconut milk (400 g)
- 1 1/2 Tsp. Sambal Olek
- 1 1/2 Tsp. salt

- 10 cherry tomatoes, halved
- A few mango cubes

NOTE: Basmati rice works well as a side dish (5 oz. gross weight per person).

**Preparation**

1. Marinate chicken in the oil, turmeric, cumin, coriander, and salt for at least 15 minutes.
2. Brown the marinated chicken in the rapeseed oil, cover, and place in oven preheated to 320°F.
3. Sautee the vegetables and garlic with a little bit of rapeseed oil in a wok skillet and add the coconut milk and bring to a boil.
4. Add Sambal Olek and salt to taste.
5. Remove chicken from oven and add to the vegetable mixture.
6. Add tomatoes and mango cubes, warm through, and season to taste.

Nutrition section contributed by Dagmar Schopen of Nutrition Counseling, Gießen, Wettenberg.

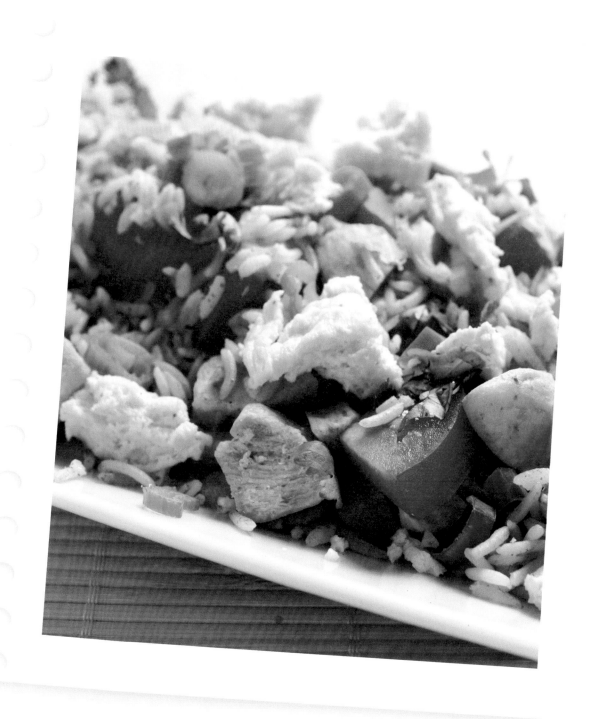

# 5 MOVEMENT IS NOT POSSIBLE WITHOUT FASCIA

The word *fascia* has only recently become popularized, some would say inappropriately so, within the field of human anatomy.

*Fascia* is defined as a sheet or band of fibrous connective tissue enveloping, separating, or binding together muscles, organs, and other tissues of the body.

The important thing to remember about fascia is that it is one type of connective tissue in a family that has many members. All fascia is connective tissue, but not all connective tissue is fascia.

There are four types of connective tissue:

1. Proper connective tissue

2. Blood

3. Bone

4. Cartilage

There are some surprising facts surrounding connective tissue, apart from the fact that blood is connective tissue and muscle isn't. The most important fact of note is that connective tissue is made up mostly of non-living material known as the extracellular matrix or ECM. This ECM is actually more important than the cells that are contained within it and make all movement and function possible.

ECM is like the inner ocean of our bodies. All the cells that we have require space around them, and this space is filled with an inert fluid that protects, cushions, and holds the cells and tissues in place. The ECM has several substances that allow for repair to take place, but its essential job is to facilitate the smooth actioning and function.

Not all ECM is the same, and it has different qualities depending on which type of cell is produced in what area of the body.

Blood, for instance, has its own type of ECM—plasma. It is the plasma that holds the red and white blood cells in place and carries them around the body. Blood is comprised of over 55% plasma and, like many connective tissues, is the forgotten yet vital component of many systems.

# 5.1 TYPES OF FASCIA

The classification of fascia is not as straightforward as we might either hope for or believe. The layer of tissue lying directly underneath the skin is known as superficial fascia (SF) and although predominantly comprised of adipose, is still a functioning fascial layer.

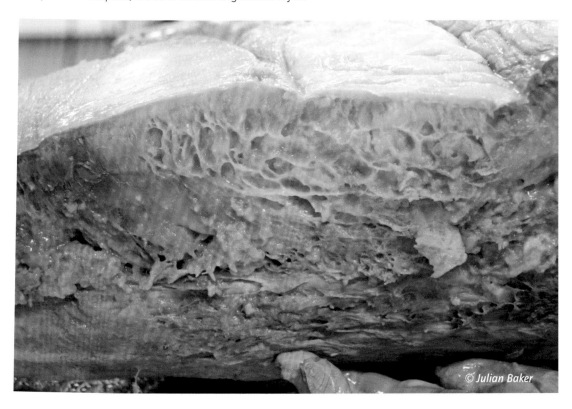

© Julian Baker

Irrespective of the amount of adipose laid down in the body, there is still a requirement for this to be held in place by a network of collagen-based fibers. This fibrous network allows for strength, movement, flexibility, and adaptation to take place, as well as for variation in adipose distribution to be supported.

The superficial layer can often be removed in one whole unit, almost like a fleecy jumpsuit, demonstrating that the tissue referred to as superficial fascia is a body-wide structure, present virtually everywhere.

Even if someone were to lose almost all their adipose tissue, the fibrous network would still be in place, visible and palpable and attached to the skin by a transparent, filmy sheath. When you pinch your skin and lift it, anywhere in the body, you are picking up not just skin, but superficial fascia. The slippery, filmy layer between these tissues and the deep fascia is what holds it in place and stops if from getting pulled off completely.

Most people in the exercise world have complicated relationships with the layer we refer to as the superficial fascia. "Can you pinch an inch?" was the phrase that was used a few years ago to suggest that perhaps you were putting on too much weight or getting flabby.

In fact, the SF plays a vital role in the stabilization of our body and is home to some interesting material, in particular a hormone called leptin.

Leptin is a hormone that regulates the fat cells in humans and also is linked to appetite. When we eat, we become full, and it is this full feeling that is driven by leptin. In obesity, the levels of leptin drop, hence the feeling of being full is harder to come by. One of the reasons that humans have become a successful species is our ability to keep taking in calories and be able to store them. Ideal in times when it was feast or famine, but not so great when we can get 24-hour fast food!

## Filmy Fascia

The layers of superficial and deep fascia, although distinct, are not separate. Instead, they slide and glide around on top of each other, but at the same time are held in place. This sliding surface has yet to be satisfactorily defined, but has been termed filmy fascia by US dissector and anatomist, Gil Hedley.

The filmy layer overlays the deep fascia and would probably be classified as a loose areolar connective tissue. It's not clear what the cellular composition of this tissue is, but studies are underway to define it's make-up, thereby making the understanding of it clearer.

## Deep Fascia

The connective tissue we call deep fascia has a different look but, in essence, is still a form of connective tissue. All fascia is made up mostly of collagen, one of the most common proteins in the body. We make collagen every day of our lives and use it both to repair our connective tissue as well as create the connections and links from one part of the system to the other.

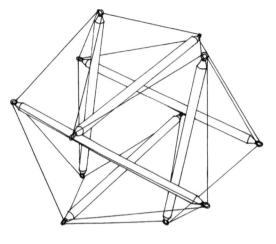

*Drawing by Bob Burkhardt*

Nature hates straight lines, and it is left to human endeavor to create firm, stable structures by piling things one on top of the other, such as bricks. In the natural world, virtually everything, from the huge to the microscopic, is curved. Curved structures not only allow for tension to be absorbed, but also to be distributed and transmitted.

Even huge, stable structures like trees are made of curved elements that will allow sway and movement to occur in strong winds and changing conditions. The human structure is no different. Collagen is a spiraled triple helix that doesn't form straight lines, but instead creates multidirectional layers that allow movement in lots of different directions.

It is also very adaptable and will lay down more fibers in a new direction of strain, if the movement and loading is repeated often enough. Collagen fibers are also responsible for repairing damaged tissue when inflammation from injury acts as a signal for the system to produce more cells.

Not all collagen fibers will be the same in terms of density, direction, or other composition, and much is dependent on the function of the individual.

One principle of understanding load mechanisms in the human form is known as bio-tensegrity, a term popularized by Steven Levin. The principle derives from the works made famous by sculptor, Kenneth Snelson, who designed tensegrity structures where solid pieces would appear to float, held in equal tension by the cords attached to them.

In much the same way, it suggests the bones of the human float in a tensional sea of connective tissue, powered by muscle and held in place by skin.

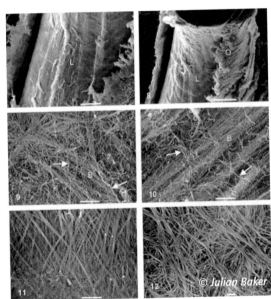

© Julian Baker

Collagen lay down is not selective and will lay down according to the instructions we give it. The fuzzy, cobweb-like structures that lie between the muscle fibers are the naturally occurring collagenous fibers that need to be there in order for normal function to take place.

In a living body, these would be wet and slippery and would create the framework for muscle to move around bone and force transmission to exist.

Muscle is the powerhouse for movement. With no muscle, the ability to lift an arm or a leg would be limited. Without fascia, it would be impossible.

Because the fascial system is continuous, it doesn't stop at the bone when the muscle does, but rather carries on across planes and in different directions, allowing what some people feel is a communicating tensional network throughout the body.

In certain areas where the connective tissue is categorized as dense and regular, the sheets of deep fascia that we see are crisscrossed and formed from fibers that travel in multiple directions.

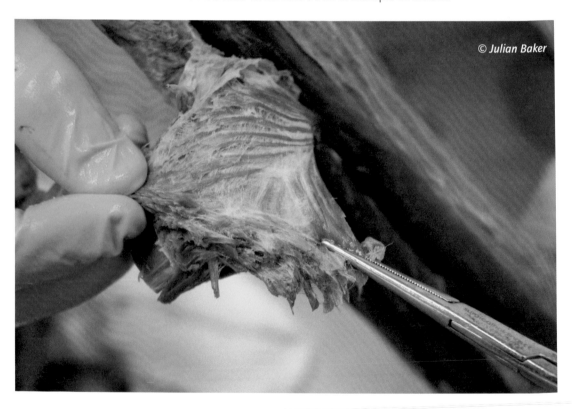

© Julian Baker

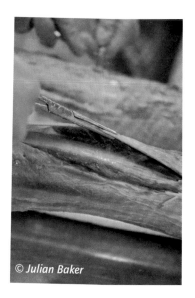

© Julian Baker

Each muscle is surrounded both by multidirectional sheets of fascia and also has fascial fibers running through and around each compartment and every muscle fiber. The integrity of muscle relies entirely on the fascia that surrounds it and holds it in place.

If fascia facilitates muscular movement, it also has the capacity to respond to lack of movement as well. As already discussed, the essential ingredient in all connective tissues is fluid in the form of ECM. Within this fluid environment live the cells that produce the collagen, fibroblasts. These cells are responding to the information given to them in order to establish what is required.

Movement, pressure, loading, and friction are all elements that will maintain the environment of the ECM. Without movement, chances are that stiffness and, thereby, lack of fluid flow will result. The outcome is the stiffness that most of us will have experienced at some stage or the other but which, if left to continue, will get worse.

An extreme example is that of Amar Bharati, a sadhu, who over 40 years ago decided to raise his arm above his head as a tribute to Shiva.

Over the years, the pain that he first experienced subsided to numbness. The collagen fibers surrounding the muscle tissue and the joint will, most probably, have become fibrous and hard. The effort of holding the arm up will have ceased to be an effort, with the fibers taking over the task of holding the arm in that position.

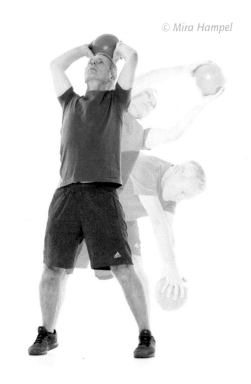

© Mira Hampel

The rest of him keeps doing a good job. We can see him squatting on the ground demonstrating great flexion ability through his knees, hips, and ankles. It's a perfect demonstration of how continued movement leads to continued ability to move and how stillness leads to stiffness.

Movement between tissues is always going to be more limited than we think. A muscle is held in place firmly by the fascia that surrounds it. Other factors come in to play as well. An arm, for instance, contains nerves that extend from the neck down to the wrist. These nerve pathways are held in place in a strictly controlled environment and have no ability or need to be able to move around in hundreds of directions. To do so would be disastrous.

Similarly, muscles slide in a relatively limited plane of movement, again held firmly in place by filmy fascia and nerve pathways. The need for movement in the human form doesn't need to rely on a model of extremes.

The treatment and stretching of fascia has attracted intense interest from the health and fitness industry over the last few years, with a myriad of "solutions" to "release" fascia that is tight, unhealthy, knotted, twisted—the list is extensive. The probability of this is that any movement, stretching, or treatment doesn't affect the fascia in that moment at all, but instead contributes to a healthier status over time.

Fascia can't be stretched in the way that a jumper can. In order to elongate tissues such as fascia, sustained pressure and lots of time are needed. The pressure, however, is probably less than originally thought as even gentle movement and tension applied over a long period will have the mechanotransduction effect already mentioned.

It was always believed that stretching was a requirement for function and that stretching the fascia was what was happening as part of deep static movements. The evidence now suggests that, in fact, stretching, while assisting in general functional movement, is not required at all as a general rule. In many instances where chronic pain is present, the advice is to stop stretching completely in order to allow function to be restored.

Neither can fascia be released. It probably doesn't need to be released in the first place as it's unlikely that the pain being caused by any issue is coming solely from the fascia. While fascia is full of nerve endings and touch receptors, pain, like movement, is a body-wide mechanism.

What fascia does need is maintenance. Daily regular movement through a wide range without extensive stretching is likely to maintain the health and flexibility of fascia well into old age. The enemy of fascia is extended bouts of stillness.

Treatment is another issue where little or no agreement has been achieved. The fascia researchers tend to come from a field where a large amount of pressure is used to achieve change, whereas the suggestion now emerging is that less pressure applied more often might have better results.

The science of fascia is still new, and there is much more work to be done before we can establish behaviors or patterns of fascial change beyond a doubt.

What is conclusive is that the watery extracellular matrix, surrounding and hydrating all our tissues, needs circulation that can only come from movement. Whatever movement means to you, keep doing it.

## About the Author

This section on fascia is contributed by Julian Baker, a leading author and speaker on the field of physical therapy and fascia. Originally from London, he has been teaching soft tissue therapies for over 25 years and has been leading human tissue dissections since 2008.

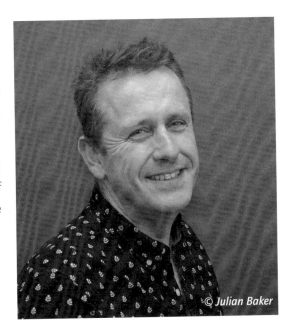
© Julian Baker

He is the author of two books on the Bowen Technique and lives in Bath in the South West of England. He leads dissection classes all over the UK. www.functionalfascia.com

# REFERENCES

Bruhn, S. & Gollhofer, A. (2001). Neurophysiologische grundlagen der propriozeption und sensomotorik. *Med. Orth. Techn., 121*, 66-71.

Deshpande, P.Y. & Patanjali. 2010. *Die Wurzeln des Yoga.* O.W. Barth Publishing.

*Seven Countries Study.* Available at www.sevencountriesstudy.com.

Swami Satyananda Saraswati. 2002. *Asana, Pranayama, Mudra and Bandha.* Yoga Publications Trust, Mungher Bihar Publisher, India.

Sivananda Yoga Centres. *Yoga.* GU Press.

Yogi Bhajan. 2009. *The Aquarian Teacher.* KRI Publisher.

# Credits

Photos:

| | |
|---|---|
| **Cover & Interior Photos:** | © Chris Kettner Fotodesign |
| **Interior Photos p. 163, 164 165, 167:** | © Adobe Stock |
| **Photos p. 18:** | From Lowery, Lamar. (2016). *Functional Fitness– The Personal Trainer's Guide,* Aachen: Meyer & Meyer, p. 20 & 21 |
| **Photos p. 10, 13, 17, 23, 28:** | Lamar Lowery |
| **Photo p. 173 (bottom):** | © Mira Hampel, www.mirahampel.de |
| **Photos from chapter 5 p. 169, 171, 172, 173, 175:** | © Julian Baker |

Design & Editing:

| | |
|---|---|
| **Cover Design:** | Sannah Inderelst |
| **Design & Layout:** | www.satzstudio-hilger.de |
| **Managing Editor:** | Elizabeth Evans |